# The Middle Manager
# in Primary Nursing

**Gloria Gilbert Mayer, R.N., Ed.D., F.A.A.N.**, received her associate degree in nursing from Miami-Dade Junior College, a B.S. from the University of Miami, an M.S. from the University of Maryland, and her M.Ed. and Ed.D. from Teachers College, Columbia University. Dr. Mayer has had a variety of professional experiences in clinical practice, administration, research, and education. She became involved in primary nursing as Associate Chief, Nursing Service for Research, at the Minneapolis Veterans Administration Medical Center, when she was evaluating the implementation and effects of primary nursing. Currently, Dr. Mayer is Senior Consultant for Health Management Systems Associates, a private consultant firm in Minneapolis, Minnesota.

**Katherine (Pam) Bailey, R.N., M.S.**, is the Associate Chief, Nursing Service for Education, at the Minneapolis Veterans Administration Medical Center. In her educational, administrative, and clinical role, she has directed the implementation of primary nursing, conducted related research, and developed a complementary educational program. Ms. Bailey received her B.S. and M.S. from the University of Minnesota. She has had experience in psychiatry, medical/surgical, and intensive care. She has taught nursing both in educational institutions and in hospitals. Prior to her current position, she was a nursing instructor at the VA.

# The Middle Manager in Primary Nursing

Gloria Gilbert Mayer, R.N., Ed.D., F.A.A.N.
Katherine Bailey, R.N., M.S.

SPRINGER PUBLISHING COMPANY
NEW YORK

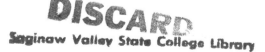

Springer Publishing Company, Inc.
200 Park Avenue South
New York, New York 10003

82 83 84 85 86 /10 9 8 7 6 5 4 3 2 1

---

**Library of Congress Cataloging in Publication Data**

Mayer, Gloria G.
　The middle manager in primary nursing.

　Bibliography: p.
　Includes index.
　1. Nursing service administration.　2. Middle managers.　I. Bailey, Katherine.　II. Title.
[DNLM: 1. Primary nursing care—Organ.　2. Administrative personnel—Nursing texts.　WY 101 M468m]
RT89.M4　　　362.1'73068　　　82-644
ISBN 0-8261-3060-7　　　AACR2
ISBN 0-8261-3061-5 (pbk.)

---

Printed in the Un

*To Tom, Kimmel, and Jeffrey;*
*Jack, Scott, Curt, and David*

# Contents

# Preface

Primary nursing is a relatively new mode of patient care delivery that is being instituted within many health care institutions around the country. This trend in delivery systems was stimulated by the recognized need to provide congruency between the philosophy and purpose of nursing services and the actual delivery of patient care by professional nurses.

The implementation of primary nursing requires role changes throughout a nursing service. Much literature addresses the roles and functions of the staff and head nurse since these are the actual care-givers within this patient-centered system. Little has been said about the upper-level manager.

The purpose of this book is to present a comprehensive examination of the role, transition, and education of the middle manager within primary nursing. The book focuses upon the transition to the system, the role of middle management, and the educational development of these individuals within primary nursing.

Since this book is specifically aimed at middle management, discussions of the role of the head and primary nurse will be limited to their relationships to the middle manager.

The contents are targeted to health care nursing personnel who are moving from traditional modes of patient care delivery to primary nursing. In addition, both undergraduate and graduate students in leadership sequences should find this book useful. Therefore it could be used as both a text and a reference book.

For the content of this book, we have drawn upon our personal professional experiences of implementing primary nursing within a large metropolitan hospital. We have developed and taught several management courses that are reflected in the contents of this book. In addition, we have participated in several research projects related to the implementation of primary nursing and have done an extensive review of current literature on the topic.

We would like to thank the many primary nurses, middle managers, and chief executives we have worked with in the process of implementing primary nursing. A special thanks to our families, who encouraged us to continue writing this book in the face of many adversities.

Gloria Mayer
Katherine Bailey

# Part I
# The Evolving Role

## EVOLUTION YIELDS NEW BIRTH

Primary nursing is a patient care delivery system which has redefined the role of the staff professional nurse. The role of the middle manager within a primary nursing setting has not been analyzed and delineated up until now. What developments led to the current role of the middle manager? What is the relationship of the middle manager to primary nursing? What needs stimulated the evolution of this role? What skills are required to meet these needs? What are the expectations and rewards of this new role?

The following chapters address these questions in relationship to primary nursing, although some of the principles presented here may be applicable to most patient-oriented delivery systems.

# Chapter 1
# Introduction to Primary Nursing

The primary goal of health care facilities is the delivery of quality patient care to the consumer. In order to accomplish this goal, a composite of various disciplines must work together to meet consumer health needs. Nursing Service, a major component contributing to this outcome, is commonly defined as the total number of individuals within an institution whose primary mission is the delivery or facilitation of nursing care to consumers.

Based upon this purpose and mission, a congruent philosophy evolves which dictates the direction and selection of a patient care delivery system. For example, if efficiency of tasks is the major focus of a service's purpose and philosophy, systems such as functional nursing are appropriate. In contrast, when a philosophy addresses meeting individualized patient needs, the selection of a nursing care modality must be congruent with this belief.

Historically, five systems of nursing care delivery have evolved. These include functional, team, case, modular, and primary modalities. These common patient care delivery systems can be compared and contrasted using several specific characteristics: major focus, accountability of individuals, lines of authority, communication patterns, assignment of personnel, and planning of patient care. (See Table 1.1 "Comparison of Patient Care Delivery Modalities.") As can be noted, functional and team

**TABLE 1.1**
**Comparison of Patient Care Delivery Modalities**

| Comparative Characteristics | Functional | Team | Case | Modular | Primary |
|---|---|---|---|---|---|
| 1. Major Focus | Complexity of tasks | Efficiency in tasks | Patient total needs | Patient total needs | Patient total needs |
| 2. Accountability | For task completion only | 8 hour task completion | Total patient care for 8 hours | 24 hours | 24 hours |
| 3. Lines of Authority | Centralized in Head Nurse | Centralized in Team Leader and Head Nurse | Centralized in Head Nurse | Decentralized to Primary Nurse | Decentralized to Primary Nurse |
| 4. Communication Patterns | Hierarchical through Head Nurse | Hierarchical through T.L. & Head Nurse | Through Head Nurse | Direct from Nurse to others | Direct from Nurse to others |
| 5. Basis of Personnel Assignments | Complexity of tasks to be accomplished | Personnel preparation & patient complexity | Complexity of total patient | Total care by Nurse based upon geographical location | Consistent total care based upon patient needs & Nurse's abilities |
| 6. Patient Care Planning | Basic data Drs. orders | Basic data, Drs. orders, nursing care plan | Basic data, Drs. orders, & individualized nursing care plan | Basic data, Drs. orders, & individualized nursing care plan | Basic data, Drs. orders, & individualized nursing care plan |

nursing modalities are similar in focus. These systems stress efficiency in the completion of tasks. In constrast, case, modular, and primary systems focus on the patient and his or her needs. Accountability of personnel varies within the systems from short-term task completion in functional nursing to 24 hour responsibility for total patient care with modular and primary nursing. The focus of authority and the patterns of communication also vary in these systems. For example, centralized authority and hierarchical communication are characteristics of functional, team, and case methods, whereas decentralized authority which encourages nonhierarchical communication patterns are advocated in modular and primary nursing. Assignments of patients to nursing personnel are based upon client needs and nursing abilities within primary nursing. In functional, team, and case methods, assignments are based upon complexity of tasks and patient's pathophysiology. Modular nursing utilizes geographical location of patients as the primary criterion for patient assignment.

The complexity and scope of patient care planning also vary among systems. Patient care planning becomes more individualized and comprehensive as the focus of each system moves toward meeting unique patient needs.

The evolution of different patient care delivery systems was based not only on nursing service philosophies but also on historical-societal and professional changes. Major stimuli to this evolution were the increased health awareness and demands by the general populace. At the same time the professional nurse achieved higher levels of education and greater role diversity. This led to an awareness that the health care systems were not meeting individualized patient needs. A movement toward a modality that focused on these needs and increased professional accountability evolved.

The primary nursing system was developed at the University of Minnesota Hospitals in the late 1960s. This system defines and describes both the type of nursing care the consumer will receive and the characteristics the nurse will possess. Primary nursing was defined by RMEC Primary Nursing Conference (1977) as the delivery of comprehensive, coordinated, continuous, and individualized total patient care through the professional nurse who has autonomy, accountability, and authority on a 24 hour basis. Under this system, the professional nurse is fully responsible for the care of several patients from the time of admission to discharge. When the primary nurse is on duty, she is always assigned to specific patients. In the absence of the primary nurse, an associate nurse follows the care plan developed by the primary nurse, thereby reinforcing continuity of care. Continuity of assignment is also encouraged for associate nurses. Documentation and verbal reporting are other means of providing continuity of patient care.

Some of the methods to insure comprehensive care include multidisciplinary planning, coordinated by the primary nurse, individualized patient assessment with a nursing care plan, and primary patient care conferences (Mayer and Bailey, 1979).

Coordination of care is the primary nurse's responsibility. This coordination involves both intradisciplinary and interdisciplinary service communication and is facilitated through the concept of decentralized communication. Documentation and verbal reporting of the patient's needs, a written plan of care, and working toward preestablished goals are examples of methods that promote coordination within primary nursing.

The nurse, through the practice of continuous, coordinated, and comprehensive care tailors the patient's care to his or her specific needs and involves the patient as well as significant others with the planning of the client's health care. This provides care uniquely designed for the specific patient, thereby creating individualized patient care.

The primary nurse should be registered and have demonstrated clinical competence. In addition, she should have the personal and professional responsibility to be knowledgeable in the nursing process, including a solid theoretical and scientific basis for action. This nurse must accept the independence inherent in autonomous practice. In addition, within primary nursing, the nurse is given the power to direct and enforce the patient's plan of care. Individually, the nurse must have the credibility to assert this kind of authority. To practice authority, the nurse must establish this power through utilization of skilled clinical, communication, and managerial competencies. Accountability implies that responsibility has been given by the system and received by the individual. Within primary nursing, a nurse assumes accountability for a given number of patients for a 24 hour period. The primary nurse demonstrates accountability through direct patient care and through verbal and written communications.

A synthesis of these qualities of primary nursing leads to a modality that addresses individualized patient needs and delivers quality care to the consumer. Quality care should be measurable based upon patient outcomes such as length of hospitalization, behavioral changes, consumer satisfaction, cost, and client involvement in health care.

Conceptually, primary nursing is interdependent upon the health care system, the consumer, and the nurse. The consumer is the recipient of individualized, coordinated, continuous, and comprehensive nursing care. The primary nurse must be an accountable practitioner with the skills required to practice with autonomy and authority. In order for the nurse to practice and the patient to receive primary nursing care, the health care system also plays a large role. This includes decentralization of communication within the system, delegation of authority, recognition of the independence of the nurse, and appropriate use of complementary resources and support systems. (See Figure 1.1, "Conceptualization of Primary Nursing.") The interface of these three interdependent elements leads to the delivery of quality patient care, which is the primary goal of any health care facility.

To implement primary nursing the delineation of the role,

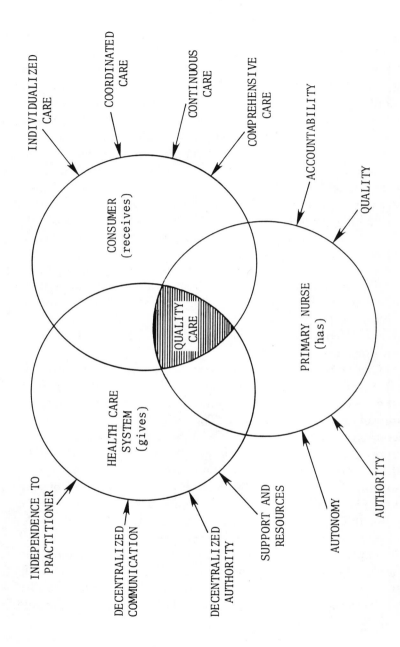

**FIGURE 1.1.** Conceptualization of primary nursing.

8

# TABLE 1.2
## Role of Primary Nurse

| | |
|---|---|
| *Definition*: | The primary nurse is a professional nurse who has accountability, authority, and autonomy for the delivery of quality nursing care for an assigned group of patients. |
| *Qualifications*: | A primary nurse is a graduate of an accredited school of nursing, is licensed to practice, and has demonstrated clinical competency in the delivery of patient care. |

*Responsibilities and Functions*:

I. The primary nurse supports the philosophy, objectives, policies, and programs of the overall nursing service.

II. The primary nurse is accountable for direct patient care to a select group of patients including the following:

  A. Identifies role in relationship to the patient and significant others.
  B. Assesses and identifies patient problems on admission and throughout hospitalization.
  C. Formulates nursing care and discharge plans based on prioritized needs and goal orientation.
  D. Communicates both verbally and in writing the proposed plan of care and movement toward problem resolution.
  E. Coordinates care with other health professionals and significant others.
  F. Delivers direct, comprehensive, safe nursing care to primary patients and selected secondary patients, including patient education.
  G. Evaluates and revises the plan of care as needed.
  H. Serves as the patient advocate through interaction with other disciplines and health care workers.
  I. Presents primary patient care conferences for purposes of staff development and communication.

III. The primary nurse is responsible for maintaining clinical and professional competence through planned and self-developmental educational programs.

functions, and responsibilities of all individuals within the system is crucial. A sample job description of a primary nurse is included as Table 1.2, "Role of Primary Nurse."

Within the health care system, the nurse manager becomes a part of one of the three elements that interface with the delivery of quality patient care. The first-line manager in most nursing services is the head nurse. The head nurse has direct contact with the consumer and the primary nurse but does not usually participate in direct patient care. If the head nurse assumes a patient caseload, she becomes a primary nurse and, therefore, a role model for other staff members.

In all instances the middle manager is a part of the health care managerial system. The middle manager is defined as the individual located on the organizational chart between the head nurse and the Director of Nursing Service. Middle managers utilize delegated authority from the top manager to plan, organize, motivate, and control subordinates toward the attainment of organizational goals. Other terms used to describe this person include *supervisor, patient care coordinator,* and *assistant director*. The term *middle manager* is used in this book to include all of these roles.

Top management usually is one or a select few individuals who are responsible for the total service. Top management assumes total accountability for nursing practice outcomes, departmental/interdisciplinary program planning, and overall service evaluation.

The selection of the primary nurse delivery system within a health care facility is dependent upon many factors. These include the philosophy of the service, the type of patient care desired, the qualifications of the nursing staff, the managerial system, and the organizational structure of the institution and service. These interdependent elements are directly related to the practice of primary nursing.

Personnel in nursing management constitute a component of the health care system. Individuals in middle management in-

teract with both the "patient care givers" and "policymakers."
Therefore, the middle manager becomes a key person to the
successful implementation and practice of primary nursing within
a health care facility. Future chapters will focus on the development of middle management and trace the evolution of its role
within primary nursing.

# Chapter 2

# Middle Management in Historical Perspective

*PATRICIA A. KOSTEN, R.N., Ed.D.*[1]

Within any well-organized health care delivery system, provision is made for nursing supervision. The evolution of the supervisory role in nursing occurred gradually and has taken various forms throughout history. In order to understand the changes in this role, a brief historical synopsis will be presented.

According to Notter and Spalding (1976), the health care of this nation was influenced by groups of women associated with nursing. Organized groups were particularly evident during the 18th and 19th centuries, when immigrants from Europe brought with them religious orders of sisters. These women, who learned nursing through the apprenticeship method, opened some of the first centers devoted exclusively to health care delivery in the United States.

The educational system that eventually developed in this country to prepare nurses in a systematic and organized manner was patterned on the Nightingale model. In her plan, Florence

[1]Patricia A. Kosten, R.N., Ed.D., is Coordinator of the Masters Program in Nursing Administration at Pace University, New York. A graduate of Seton Hall's baccalaureate program in nursing, she received her master's and doctorate at Teachers College, Columbia University. She has had many years of nursing experience at all levels. For the past decade she has been engaged in nursing education, focusing mainly on administration, and has maintained a small private practice.

Nightingale provided for the supervisory, management, and leadership development of nursing students through extensive clinical practice. Two types of preparation were designated—one for the general nurse, who had one year's training followed by three years of supervised practice. The second type of nurse was prepared to serve on a staff of teachers and had one year's training and two years of supervised practice. Miss Nightingale maintained that the place for the student to learn was at the bedside. "She urged the ward sister to 'learn the student' and to plan for her instruction." (Notter and Spalding, 1976, p. 14). This individualized learning, tailored to the specific needs of a given student, is a reputable mode of education. Although the apprenticeship method has its limitations, today we are quite cognizant of the merits of learning from the experienced practitioner. One can readily imagine the nurse neophyte emulating the management behaviors of her teacher. Opportunities for her to practice these newly acquired skills were no doubt available to some extent.

The first schools founded in the United States were established in 1873 at the Bellevue Training School in New York City, The Connecticut Training School in New Haven, and the Boston Training School (later the Massachusetts General Training School) in Boston. These were patterned after the Nightingale system and at the start were supported by a few physicians, but were generally opposed by the medical profession.

Opposition from medicine seemed to stem from divergence of opinion about control rather than from rejection of the concept of education for nursing. As early as 1869 a committee of the American Medical Association members urged the organization to take the leadership in developing a system of education for nurses. They recommended that hospital schools be under the direction of the physician and presented an outline of areas of teaching and the duties of nurses (Lambertsen, 1958).

These training programs are described by Lambertsen (1958):

[Student] assignments depended on facilities available and services needed. The first programs were one year in length, but it was found that by extending the course to two years students could be utilized as head nurses. Experience in patient care was provided in the first year and the second year was concerned with ward administration [p. 13].

In both the 19th and early 20th centuries, the general focus of nursing education was that one learned by doing. This was reflected in the preparation of both clinical practitioners and nursing educators. The type of managerial experience provided for the student of this period was on-the-job training through assumption of head nurse responsibilities. Undoubtedly, such a system had some undesirable outcomes because it was dependent upon rote learning. In a historical analysis, this method of education can be considered an "experiment" in learning the management process. Today, in the educational programs, application of the management process occurs first in controlled laboratory settings with simulated situations, whereas the former is "real life in action."

Historically, a transition occurred in the educational preparation of nurses at the turn of the century. Some colleges took the initiative to modify the on-the-job training approach to nursing education by providing formal courses. As early as 1899, Teachers College, Columbia University, New York, offered a course of studies for nurses wishing to prepare for school and hospital administration (Dolan, 1978). These studies, entitled "Hospital Economics Course," were one year in length and were offered in the Department of Domestic Science (Christy, 1969). Special courses dealing with hospital and training school management were developed, taught, and financed by the American Society of Superintendents of Training Schools for Nurses under the leadership of Isabel Hampton Robb. Study of psychology, science, household economics, and biology were part of the course and were offered to nurses through existing courses in these subjects at Teachers College.

This course of study was extended to a two-year program in 1905 and included special lectures on hospital administration, working essentials, and hospital construction, hospital laundry, and hospital planning.   Christy quotes from the 1907–1908 Teachers College bulletin (1969):

> The two-year curriculum totaled 60 points: 12 of General and Educational Psychology; 30 in Hospital Economics, School Hygiene, Biology and Domestic Science; and 18 in electives such as Chemistry, Bacteriology, Geography, English and Physical Education [p. 36].

As hospital programs increased in number, nurse educators organized and developed standards for a school curriculum.   In 1917 the Committee on Education of the National League of Nursing Education prepared a public document in which they identified those elements that composed acceptable educational preparation of nurses (NLN, 1917).   Interest during this period was also directed to collegiate preparation for the nurse.   The first program opened at University of Minnesota in 1909, and this was followed seven years later in New York by a joint program of the Schools of Nursing at the Presbyterian Hospital and Teachers College, Columbia University.   While the former has continued until the present time, the latter endured only until 1924 (Lambertsen, 1958, p. 22).

During the 1920s increasing numbers of university-conducted schools of nursing emerged, directed by graduates of Teachers College (Christy, 1969, p. 79).   By 1935 course offerings were increased to:

> . . . ten areas in which a nurse could major: Teaching in Schools of Nursing, Supervision in Schools of Nursing, Administration in Schools of Nursing, Administration in Hospitals, Public Health Nursing, Teaching in Public Health, Teaching of Home Nursing and Child Care, and Nursing and Health Education [Christy, 1969, p. 81].

The areas of the supervision major provided formalized approaches to management of personnel and equipment, control of supply utilization, and plant maintenance.

At a conference held at Teachers College in January 1933,

the decision was made to form an association of Collegiate Schools of Nursing. Lambertsen (1958) states:

> The purposes of this organization were to develop nursing education on a professional and collegiate level, to promote and strengthen relationships between schools of nursing and institutions of higher education and to promote study and experimentations in nursing service and nursing education [p. 22].

Prior to 1930 the notion that clinical learning alone constituted adequate nursing education was prevalent. It was during this decade that both classroom and clinical practice emerged in nursing education and dual positions of supervisor/instructor were developed.

In most hospital programs education was the responsibility of the director of nursing, and head nurses and supervisors provided both classroom and clinical instruction. As one might expect, the decision to provide education, when service needs were pressing, was difficult to make. As the result, student learning was set aside as a lesser priority.

The importance of clinical learning as an essential component of nursing education was consistently upheld by nursing educators through the National League of Nursing Education (1927):

> Students should be impressed with the fact that the ward is a place for study just as much as the classroom or library and every effort should be made to connect the teaching in the ward with that of the classroom and vice versa [p. 52].

It was also during the period of the late 1920s and early 1930s that one began to see the beginnings of nursing research. Isabel M. Steward, of Teachers College, was greatly impressed by the results of the time and motion studies for improvement of efficiency and home economics and saw their potential application to nursing. Miss Steward was prompted to study and apply these techniques to nursing (Christy, 1969, pp. 78, 79).

With the economic pressures of the Great Depression many private duty nurses sought employment in hospitals. Since student nurses provided the major portion of the nursing staff, competition for staff positions was great. Although the employment of experienced practitioners would seem to have been a desirable addition to the nursing service of the hospital and provided potential role models for students, directors were vocal in their objections to the employment of these co-professionals. They said they resented criticism, were difficult to discipline and extravagant in the use of supplies, increased the cost of nursing services to the hospital, and were unpredictable in their length of employment. On the other hand, graduate nurses also had many objections to hospital employment, which included the inability to plan and give patients the care based on needs, and the lack of recognition and dignity attributed to their service (NLNE, 1933, p. 14).

Historically some attributed this attitude to military influences because during the Spanish American War nurses held no rank and were therefore subject to commands of the less qualified (Dolan, 1978, p. 291). This situation was corrected to some extent during World War I, but many examples of militaristic behavior were still present, such as student line-ups for inspection before reporting for duty and standing at attention when addressed by a supervisor or physician.

One serious effect of this type of influence was the promotion of unquestioning obedience to one's superior. The role of the nurse was influenced both by society's concept of the role of a woman in a male dominant culture and the trait of subservience as an ethical and moral strength. Nurses' feelings of inferiority, lack of sense of professional self, and inadequately developed ego strength handicapped the professional development of nursing well into the present era.

During and following World War II, numbers and qualities of auxiliary nursing personnel increased. Functions previously performed exclusively by nurses were undertaken by practical nurses, nurses aides, orderlies, and corpsmen. For this category of personnel to function most effectively, the nurse assumed the responsibility of organizing, delegating, and supervising their own work. Classroom preparation of the student nurse for this new role was nonexistent. Once more, nursing reverted back to the Nightingale model, the apprenticeship on-the-job training, in order to develop the supervisory potential of the beginning nurse.

Hospital nursing programs continued to provide nursing services in exchange for educational experiences for students. Managerially, it was not unusual for students to assume complete responsibility for hospital wards during evening and night tours of duty. Their sole source of supervision was the evening/night supervisor who had responsibility for the entire hospital.

As medical science advanced, nurses began to assume new responsibilities for patient care, such as drug administration and treatments. Nurses recognized their need for preparation in organization and management as these responsibilities increased and the nursing service structures became more complex (Yura, Ozimek, and Walsh, 1976, pp. 6–7).

During the 1950s greater emphasis was placed on the preparation of nurses for supervisory positions at all levels (Miller, 1968). Specific ways cited by the Committee on the Functions of Nursing (1948) in which the nurse needed to exercise this leadership in her own profession included "improving those nursing skills already in existence and developing new nursing skills; in teaching and supervising other nurses and auxiliary workers . . ." (p. lx). Graduate programs offering a master's degree in specialty areas and a functional major in nursing administration were developed throughout the country. These programs obviously met a portion of the need. Still, the vast majority of diploma and baccalaureate graduates received no formalized educational preparation in supervision, yet were filling these positions in hospitals and other health care agencies.

Most of the leadership behavior was learned on the job, through the apprenticeship system and by trial and error.

Although this type of preparation was inadequate, many fine managers evolved. Yura et al. (1976) state:

> However, many nurses were lost to the profession because of their frustration in having responsibilities thrust upon them that they had not been prepared to meet through education or experience [p. 7].

Baccalaureate programs of nursing received great impetus during this period. As they strengthened, the dichotomy between collegiate education and diploma nursing preparation became more pronounced (Dolan, 1978, p. 314). Under the leadership of Professor R. Louise McManess of Teachers College, a committee undertook the study of levels of function within nursing. Conceptualizing the functions of nursing within a spectrum, Professor McManess envisioned a wide range. The spectrum involved performance of skills of varying complexity extending on a continuum from the simple to the highly complex (Teachers College, 1948).

This proposal was developed in a study by Dr. Mildred Montag (1951) in her doctoral dissertation. Dr. Montag believed that programs could be developed in agencies and educational institutions to prepare persons to perform functions at the furthest end of the spectrum—the less complex functions. Functions of intermediate complexity would require technical training in the college setting, and highly complex functions would require professional nursing preparation (at the baccalaureate level).

The associate degree programs that eventually were established as a result of Dr. Montag's work were intended to be terminal programs. "Montag proposed that the graduate of an associate degree nursing program function mainly by implementing the decisions of persons more expertly prepared and experienced in nursing (Dolan, 1978, p. 316)." This reflected the expectation that the professional nurse (the baccalaureate graduate) would not only possess the ability to intervene in highly complex nursing situations, but would also be able to managerially direct the less qualified nurse technician.

Even today, formal baccalaureate preparation for this kind of supervision is usually not readily identifiable in nursing curricula. The concept of leadership is given some consideration from a theoretical point of view. Some nursing programs do, however, provide clinical experiences in which students assume responsibility for patient care coordination. To direct others the nurse must possess some leadership ability as identified by Yura et al. (1976):

> Nursing leadership is a process whereby a person who is a nurse affects the actions of others in goal determination and achievement. This implies the defining and planning for nursing in an interactional setting [p. 93].

In contrast, current nursing programs aim to develop certain intellectual skills needed for leadership. Skills such as critical thinking, problem solving, making sound judgments, validating inferences, and predicting the success of solutions are incorporated in some present-day programs. In addition, extensive focus is given to interpersonal relationships, human behavior, communication techniques, and group process.

In general, however, little or no provision is made for learning the management process within the hospital setting. Many of the needs for the development of potential head nurses and supervisors are met through post-baccalaureate programs. On-the-job training is still widely relied upon and is reinforced through in-service education programs. Enrollment in master's programs in nursing administration is many times the preparation of choice.

## SUMMARY

Strides in the development of sound educational preparation for the nurse are evident in the review of the history of nursing in the United States. Significant advances toward a professional status that is recognized by society at large have been made.

Management needs in the delivery of nursing care within the hospital nursing service have become more pronounced as secondary and tertiary intervention become more complex. The stated purpose of baccalaureate nursing programs is to prepare first level practitioners—those who will initially function under supervision. The assumption is that graduate education is the formal preparatory route for the potential nurse manager.

It is common practice, nonetheless, to promote nurses to these supervisory positions without this advanced academic preparation. Since the management/supervisory preparation of the baccalaureate graduate for this reality is relatively nonexistent in preservice preparation, hospitals have met this need in other ways. On-the-job training and well conducted in-service educational programs have made significant contributions to this endeavor and have had successful results.

# Chapter 3
# Primary Nursing: Theoretical Model of Management

The nursing managers' primary responsibility is patient care.
—Byers and Klink (1978, p. 120)

## INTRODUCTION

The role of the nursing supervisor, whatever the official title, is often the most ill-defined role in the hospital hierarchy
—Stevens (1974, p. 37)

A clear middle managerial role is essential for a dynamic and effective nursing service. Differentiating this role is often difficult because traditionally it has been thought of as an expanded head nurse's role. Prior to defining this role, one must analyze the multivariables that have impact on this position. Figure 3.1, "Variables Having Impact on the Middle Managerial Role," defines these variables and includes consumer demands, professional standards, organizational structure, and educational preparation of the individual.

Today nursing practice has theoretically evolved into a pa-

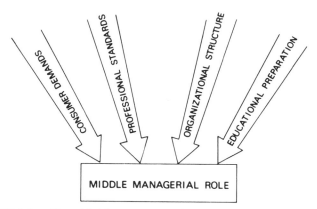

**FIGURE 3.1.** Variables having impact on the middle managerial role.

tient-centered service responsive to consumer needs and demands, and, therefore, the patient is the focus of all activities. In order to make this focus a reality, all individuals within the health care configuration must be sensitive to the recipient's needs. This becomes even more crucial in a competitive health care system, where the consumer is knowledgeable concerning his own health.

A consumer-centered philosophy is exemplified through the utilization of professional standards, which includes the nursing process and adapts the problem solving technique to patient care delivery. The nursing process consists of assessment, patient care planning, implementation, and evaluation. This process has an impact on and a relevancy for the middle manager's role in nursing. Generally, the literature addresses the nursing process in relationship to direct patient care. However, this process is equally applicable for the middle manager, who usually delivers patient care indirectly. There is heavy correlation between the nursing process and the management process. The management process involves planning/organizing, motivating/directing, and evaluating/controlling.

Within the organization, the patient-centered concept must

also be reflected. This is usually stated through the philosophy and objectives of the service and becomes operational through the patient care delivery system. Primary nursing is the patient-centered system that is currently being advocated. This patient care delivery system emphasizes different components within the managerial role, including skills, techniques, methods, and the utilization of the managerial process. Therefore, traditional methods of management are not appropriate when addressing a client-oriented system.

## CONCEPTUALIZATION

In client-oriented health care delivery, a unique relationship exists between the individual and the system. When the consumer is well the system acts as a potential support. Whether it is the physician in the clinic, the dietitician, or the nurse, this system is available to the consumer for use as needed.

Graphically, this relationship between the client and the health care system is illustrated by an umbrella. The handle and spokes of the umbrella represent the health care system, the spokes specifically representing the multifacets of the health care organization. The fabric of the umbrella represents the most important part of the relationship, the client. When the umbrella is closed, the client is not actively utilizing the system. This concept is illustrated in Figure 3.2, "Relationship Between Consumer and Health Care System."

As the individual moves along the continuum of health, the umbrella opens and provides specific resources and services to the client. Figure 3.3, "Supportive Elements of the Health Care System," represents this conceptualization. In this figure the spokes portray a few of the disciplines within the health care system which may support the client in meeting his health care needs.

Management within each discipline consists of many differ-

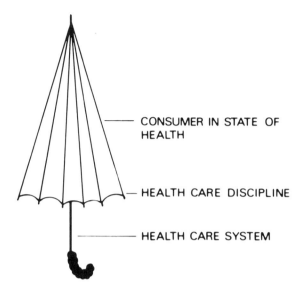

**FIGURE 3.2.**   Relationship between consumer and the health care system.

ent and varied roles. "Role" is defined as that specific behavioral criterion that defines how an individual within a given position should act in both lateral and vertical associations and interactions. To actualize a specific role two basic components are essential: cognitive knowledge and observable application of theory. Cognitive knowledge and observable behavior within each discipline utilize basic principles common to all services—principles of the management process. However, the emphasis in the process varies dependent upon the philosophy and organization of the health care system. For example, if the system focuses primarily on cost effectiveness and budgetary restraints, emphasis within the components of the process will be geared in that direction. If there is a combined focus on quality patient care and cost effectiveness, negotiation and compromise will be emphasized to achieve both components.

Within nursing service one of the elements that dictates

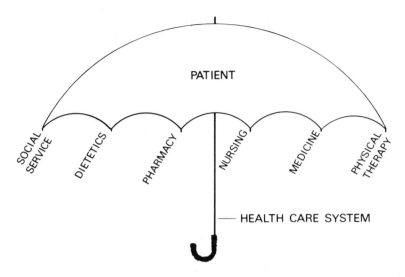

**FIGURE 3.3.**    Supportive elements of the health care system.

process component emphasis is the delivery system selected. It is within these systems that roles evolve. The specific types of roles are dependent on the association and relationship within the total organization and the mode of patient care delivery selected by the service.

The role most often addressed in literature is that of the primary nurse. The primary nurse is in closest proximity to the patient. It is the primary nurse who is accountable for the coordination, individualization, and comprehensiveness of direct patient care.

Other individual roles within nursing service complement the primary nurse. These individuals interact with the patient but in an indirect manner. For example, the first-line manager, the head nurse, may elect to be a primary nurse under specific circumstances and, therefore, have direct patient interaction. In other situations, the head nurse may be a support and resource to the primary nurse. Therefore, this first-line management role may be a patient care planner and deliverer or a consultant and/or teacher.

The role of top management is represented in the organizational chart by the director/administrator of nursing service. Within this managerial position, patient care is effected indirectly through the interactions with other professionals.

The role of the middle manager is between top and first-line management in the formal organizational structure. The middle manager is commonly entitled the "clinical supervisor" or "coordinator" and is directly responsible to the Director of Nursing Service or her designee. In middle managerial roles responsibilities to the patient are also of an indirect nature. However, it is important to continue the client-centered focus.

In Figure 3.4, "Nursing Service Organization Within Pri-

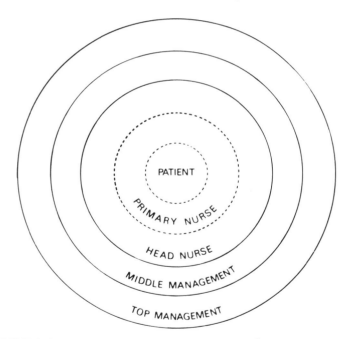

**FIGURE 3.4.** Nursing service organization within primary nursing.

mary Nursing," the patient is the center and the focus of all activities. The primary nurse is the closest to the patient followed by the head nurse, middle, and then top management. Within this configuration, the solid lines represent an artificial separation from the patient. Any one of these layers may be removed and/or bypassed from the system. For example, in some primary nursing models, the role of the first-line and middle manager is combined into one position.

In order to retain a client-centered system within primary nursing, unique relationships must be developed and retained among personnel organizationally above and below the middle manager. These relationships include those of consultation, cooperation, coordination, collaboration, evaluation, and direction. Traditionally, in managerial literature, these are described as staff and line relationships.

The middle manager's role must be defined and delineated professionally and organizationally based upon the relationship to staff and to the patient. Development of skills to effectively and efficiently demonstrate a patient-centered managerial position must be accomplished.

Subsequent chapters will deal with the skills, techniques, and methods used to implement the management process in a middle managerial role within a client-centered primary nursing system.

# Chapter 4
# Needs That Determine the Middle Managerial Role

## INTRODUCTION

Roles within a health care delivery system evolve to meet the needs of the individuals within the structure. As discussed in the previous chapter, several variables have impact on the middle managerial role. This chapter will explore two of these variables: the consumer, and some of the elements within an organizational structure.

Patient care delivery models demand role changes, and one role within primary nursing is that of the middle manager. What are the factors within primary nursing that have stimulated the middle manager's role change? Various groups of individuals with specific needs have promoted the change in the middle manager's role. The patient is the individual primarily responsible for providing the stimuli for this evolution. Additional groups and individuals within the organization that play an important part in the determination of the role, functions, and responsibilities of the middle manager include the nursing service in totality, and such persons as top management, middle managerial peers, the head

nurse, and the primary nurse. A discussion of the needs of each
individual and/or group that have impact on the middle managerial role will follow.

## NEEDS OF THE PATIENT

When a patient is admitted into a hospital, he or she seeks some
type of health care assistance. With this in view, several patient
needs can be identified that directly impinge upon the role of the
middle manager. These include the need for:

1. Direct patient care delivered by a qualified staff,
2. A safe environment, and
3. Coordinated health care and accessibility to total hospital
   services.

To fulfill the patient's need for quality nursing care, the
selection of an appropriate staff is the responsibility of the middle
manager. In the selection of such a staff, education, skills, and
experience are important. The ability to make this selection
requires that the middle manager be able to identify the needs of
the patients within her area. Second, the middle manager must
readily assess the education, competency, and experience levels
of nurse applicants and staff members. Last, the middle manager
must assure congruency between the patients' needs and the
nurses' qualifications. In the correlation of these components, the
role of the middle manager becomes more patient-centered.

Once the middle manager selects qualified personnel with
the abilities to meet client needs, this staff must then be allocated
to patient care units according to priorities. These patient priorities are based upon needs within the entire hospital rather than
on specific units. Since the middle manager is the person who has
the total evaluation of the service, she is the only one who can
make these decisions.

A second patient need is that of a safe environment, which

relates to equipment, supplies, and safe surroundings. These are all within the jurisdiction of the middle manager. All patient care systems demand a safe environment, but primary nursing requires special attention to environmental factors that promote the concept. Examples of these include supplies that facilitate and coordinate continuity of patient care, such as bulletin boards for assignments and provisions for bedside documentation. Detailed procedures outlining accepted practice criteria and promoting access to equipment allow the nurse to use her time wisely, therefore increasing direct patient care contacts.

Another environmental factor is the actual selection and evaluation of equipment used in patient care. The ability to establish valid criteria upon which equipment may be evaluated for safety contributes heavily to patient well-being.

Another patient need that the middle manager must satisfy is the need for hospital services and resources. In a complex health care facility, the middle manager must be aware of the multiplicity of the services available and the procedures required to activate them. The middle manager serves as a resource and facilitator to meet this patient need.

Because the role of the middle manager within primary nursing evolves primarily from patient needs, the functions and responsibilities will vary as patients' needs change.

Additional variables that affect the middle manager are elements of an organizational structure. At the present time the organizational structure generally characteristic of hospitals and nursing service is that of a hierarchical-classical organization (Schultz and Johnson, 1976, p. 151). Within this hierarchical formal organization, the administrative process has the potential to develop to newer and greater dimensions such as those within primary nursing. Supervisory positions within a hierarchical structure are numerically determined by such factors as total number of nursing units within the hospital. Instances in which directors of nursing service have superseded supervisory positions and head nurses report directly to the directors have had varying rates of success. The need for the middle manager is generally seen as a necessity within the complex hospital organization. Where authority is placed and when and by whom power is used within an organization are dependent upon several factors:

1. The number of levels inherent in the organization,
2. The extent to which authority and power are delegated in conjunction with responsibility,
3. The effectiveness of decision making, and
4. The acceptability of decisions by persons at the lowest hierarchical level (Yura et al., 1976, p. 73).

The individual within the organizational structure of the nursing service department of the hospital affects and is affected by it. Therefore, understanding the organization and how it functions is essential to nursing supervision. Knowing the philosophy, purposes, and objectives of the nursing service department enables the supervisor to envision how patient care can best be delivered. Knowledge of the mechanism for problem solving, provided in the department's formal structure, is also essential. The mode of patient care delivery, which makes the structure operational, has impact on the individuals within the organization. Roles are created by being sensitive to the needs of these groups of individuals. The discussion which follows will focus on some of the needs of these groups of individuals that have the potential for satisfaction through the skills of the middle manager.

## NEEDS OF THE PRIMARY NURSE

Since the patient is the core of primary nursing and the individual within the institution who is closest to the client is the primary nurse, the needs of this nurse are crucial in the determination of the middle manager's role. What are the needs of the primary nurse?

The major need of the primary nurse that can be fulfilled within the middle managerial role is the promotion and facilitation of overall structural change. The middle manager within the hierarchical structure of the organization has the power and authority to make these types of changes. Examples include:

1. Obtaining equipment necessary for model implementation,
2. Initiating and promoting organizational changes such as policies and procedures, roles, functions, and responsibilities, and
3. Selecting and scheduling personnel to meet patient needs.

A second need is that of a communicative link to and from top management. In a large organization, the middle manager serves as a direct link to communicate with and obtain feedback from top management regarding selected issues. Types of communication that illustrate this pattern include those related to patient status and incidences, proposed changes in policies and procedures, and administrative issues. This need for communication can be made verbally or in written form.

Another need of the primary nurse is that of a clinical, managerial, and resource consultant. Under normal circumstances the head nurse serves in this role; however, in complex, unique situations the primary nurse may require advice and affirmation of decisions from an individual higher in the organization. An example of this is in the use of a nontraditional or experimental patient care intervention.

## NEEDS OF THE HEAD NURSE

The head nurse is another individual within the organization who dictates the role of the middle manager. His or her needs can be categorized into the following areas:

1. Guidance in administrative and unit organization,
2. Assistance in staff development and related programs, and
3. Consultation and resource expertise.

Administratively, the head nurse needs:

1. Assistance in the development and implementation of unit level objectives,
2. Guidance in application of time management, and
3. Consultation in problem solving.

It is the middle manager who assists the head nurse in correlating unit level objectives with those of the total nursing service. These should reflect the philosophy, current status, and future directions of the overall nursing service primary nursing model. This correlation lends credence and continuity to overall nursing service endeavors.

The effective use of the principles of time management is another head nurse administrative skill that requires middle management assistance. Primary nursing requires a large time commitment from the head nurse, and, therefore, middle managers must assist the head nurse in allocating time aimed at clinical activities. Middle managers must be selective in the utilization of the head nurse's time off the unit. Activities off the unit should focus on relevant issues related to clinical practice and effective use of primary nurses. In addition, the head nurse requires guidance in the distribution of time related to unit activities.

Traditionally, supervisors encourage the active phase of the management process rather than the planning aspect. In primary nursing the head nurse needs to be allowed time to accomplish planning of evaluative activities, such as performance evaluation and audits.

Another aspect requiring middle management assistance is related to the allocation of staff time. The head nurse needs guidance in the planning of overall staffing patterns and tours of duty and in selecting floating personnel, in order to promote the concept of continuity within primary nursing.

Finally, the head nurse administratively needs consultation related to problem solving. In many instances the head nurse needs assistance in identification of problems based on data analysis. Problem resolution requires selection of the best alternative. Discussions related to alternative solutions with a supervisor vindicate or invalidate a potential mode of resolution.

Another major need of the head nurse is assistance in staff development and related programs. This assistance may be related to ward and centralized orientation and in-service, improvement of staff performance, and personal professional growth.

The "backbone" of the development of a primary nurse is a solid orientation program. This involves a high correlation between classroom and ward experience, plus tutelage to meet individual needs. The head nurse or designee is responsible for this orientation, but effectively fulfilling this developmental role may be superseded by patient care needs. When such conflicts occur, the middle manager must intervene because she has greater resources available.

A high correlation must also exist between ward and centralized in-service programs. Frequently, head nurses need assistance in correlating staff development programs with overall quality assurance data, such as audit findings, infection control statistics, turnover studies, time and motion studies, and incidence reports. Head nurses also need guidance in implementing follow-up corrective actions related to deficits in patient care delivery.

The head nurse requires assistance in promoting staff performance. This includes the motivation of superior and average performers and the remedial development of those demonstrating deficits. The middle manager is a resource in the development of the head nurse in this area. Likewise, head nurses require assistance in the development of potential leaders among the ward personnel.

Finally, the head nurse needs a managerial role model to actively demonstrate utilization of the management process within and congruent with the concept and principles of primary nursing in order to develop personally and professionally as a head nurse in a primary nurse model. The head nurse also requires an available resource to provide consultation in a variety of areas, including those related to patient care, staff, and the implementation of new programs and the closure of old ones. One such example is the implementation of primary nursing at the ward level. In this situation, the middle manager must demonstrate support to the head nurse, provide necessary tools and staffing, and allow growth of the first-line manager and ward staff.

Another area where consultation is needed is when a crisis arises. This is a flexible task and responsibility since the needs and the circumstances vary. However, the availability of ready consultation is crucial to the safe operation of the unit.

## NEEDS OF MIDDLE MANAGERIAL PEERS

In primary nursing, the middle managerial peer group also has needs that influence the role. These needs can be classified into two categories: (1) peer support within the role and (2) evaluation.

The need for peer support can be satisfied through group participation in activities such as the sharing of new methods and ideas, problem solving, brainstorming, cooperative long- and short-term planning, and assistance in the time of crisis. Cooperation with overall nursing service staffing is crucial to the development and maintenance of an effective patient care delivery system.

A second need of middle managerial peers is related to evaluation. Discussion and consultation related to the middle managerial role and evaluation of nursing care delivered by the entire service are examples of validation that may be done by second-line supervisors. This is crucial in long-range planning, which is an integral task of middle management.

## NEEDS OF THE NURSING SERVICE AND TOP MANAGEMENT

The middle manager needs to be responsive to the overall goals of nursing service and top management. Examples of goals requiring middle managerial attention include:

1. Maintenance of an organizational structure,
2. Facilitation of quality patient care,
3. Evaluation of patient outcomes,
4. Maintenance of a cost effective service,
5. Interaction and effective utilization of support services and other disciplines, and
6. Maintenance of employee morale and job satisfaction.

The mission and philosophy of nursing service dictate the directions and organization of the department. The top manager is responsible for insuring that the mission is accomplished and the philosophy implemented. This is conceptualized and planned at the top management level and delegated to middle management for purposes of actualization. Therefore, top management requires that the middle manager implement the philosophy and objectives through the organizational structure and assist in related long-term planning.

Through the middle manager, top management insures quality of patient care. Top management requires that the middle manager have the skills to institute and maintain such a delivery system, which promotes individualized, comprehensive, continuous, and coordinated total patient care.

Quality of care must be evaluated both externally and internally. Standards set forth by external organizations such as the American Nurses' Association and the Joint Commission for Accreditation of Hospitals may be the basis for external review. Internally, a program that includes a comprehensive, integrated, evaluative program must be operational. Audits, safety incident reports, and medication errors serve as a basis for patient care evaluation, and it is through the middle managers that top management accomplishes corrective actions.

Top management needs patient care delivery within a cost effective framework. For example, baccalaureate and associate degree registered nurses, LPNs, and Nursing Assistants must be distributed to insure that the concepts of primary nursing can be achieved in an efficient manner. Within primary nursing, top management needs a coordinator to insure productive interaction and utilization of support services and other disciplines. This is accomplished through the middle manager who oversees and consults with the primary nurse in the use of these services.

The maintenance of employee morale and job satisfaction are crucial elements to insure a stabilized, productive, and creative nursing service. The middle manager interacts with the staff, assesses the psychological climate, and is in a position of authority to make changes to promote staff well-being.

# Chapter 5

# Skills Required by the Middle Manager within Primary Nursing

Unmet needs within individuals in a given environment stimulate the creation of new roles. Analysis of a role leads to the identification of skills required within a position. In the middle manager's role, skills are required which focus both on the managerial aspects of patient care and on the personnel who deliver that care. Such skills are not unique to primary nursing and are found in all types of nursing management; however, the emphasis on specific skill categories varies. This variance occurs because goals of specific patient care delivery modalities differ. In primary nursing the central focus of all goals is the patient.

Managerial skills can be divided into three general areas: (1) technical skills, (2) those related to human interactions, and (3) conceptualization. A few examples of technical skills include: manual manipulation, interpretation of data, and time scheduling. Human interaction skills deal with one's ability to communicate effectively, interpret messages, and give appropriate feedback. The ability to conceptualize includes problem solving, goal setting, and establishment of action plans. All skills required of the middle manager within primary nursing include the above areas. The discussion that follows includes skills that must be developed at a sophisticated level within primary nursing:

1. Application of cognitive knowledge,
2. Utilization of the management process,
3. Communication effectiveness,
4. Application of teaching and learning principles,
5. Utilization of change principles,
6. Implementation,
7. Evaluation, and
8. Interaction with organized labor.

## APPLICATION OF COGNITIVE KNOWLEDGE

There are four areas of cognitive knowledge that are essential for application within the primary nursing middle manager's role. These are related to clinical skills, the managerial process, the concept of primary nursing, and professional trends. For the middle manager to obtain this type of cognitive knowledge, motivation is crucial because it requires personal effort. This knowledge can be obtained by reading current literature, viewing audiovisual materials, attending appropriate educational offerings, and conferring with knowledgeable consultants.

Traditionally, skills of clinical practice are taught in nursing education. Expertise in these skills are a qualification of the primary nurse role. In traditional patient care delivery systems, the need for clinical expertise decreases as one advances in the organizational hierarchy; however, this is not true in primary nursing. Nursing process and technical and therapeutic relationship skills must be retained in a managerial role within a system that focuses on the patient.

The application of these skills is important because it establishes the credibility of the middle manager clinically and, therefore, facilitates the consultative role. For example, as a resource person, the middle manager must be able to assist in the identification of complex patient problems, propose creative alternatives, and demonstrate new techniques and skills for problem resolution. It is extremely difficult for an individual who is in management to retain these clinical skills; therefore, a deliberate effort must be made to maintain these competencies.

In addition to clinical competence, application of the management process is essential. This includes the theory of management, organizational structure, and the philosophy, policy, and procedures of the individual health care agency. This theoretical knowledge can be acquired through formal education or within organizational development programs. The material related to a particular organization can be reviewed in the health care agency's documents. Further discussion of the management process will be found under the appropriate heading in this chapter.

A third category of cognitive knowledge required of the middle manager is a theoretical and pragmatic understanding of the concept of primary nursing. This involves an analysis of the concept and identification of the essential components that promote comprehensive, coordinated, continuous, individualized total patient care. These crucial components can be demonstrated in nursing care planning, documenting, continuity of daily assignments, decentralized communication patterns, patient care conferences, and 24-hour accountability. Following comprehension of the basic concept, the middle manager must analyze her role within this delivery system and make the two elements congruent with the other. Knowledge of primary nursing can be obtained through a literature review, formal educational and clinical experiences, and consultation.

The implementation process of primary nursing also requires cognitive understanding by the middle manager. This includes a working knowledge of each step and phase, plus the skill to assess and evaluate progress. The current literature minimally assists or guides the middle manager in acquiring knowledge. Therefore, resources, such as consultants and/or preceptorships with individuals who have implemented the concept, become imperative. Visits to units practicing primary nursing are useful. Because no one method of implementation has been identified as most appropriate, the middle manager must be creative and adapt the implementation process of other settings to her own situation.

A knowledge of professional trends is also required by the primary nurse middle manager. This knowledge aids the middle manager in goal setting, avoiding pitfalls, and determining policies related to primary nursing. Knowledge of trends helps the middle manager to avoid obsolescence prior to implementation.

## UTILIZATION OF THE MANAGEMENT PROCESS

A second skill required of the middle manager within primary nursing is the ability to carry out the management process. For the purposes of definition, the management process includes skills of planning and organizing, motivating and directing, and controlling. It is through this process that the goals of nursing service are met. Within this process, the middle manager brings together resources to perform a service or create a product, and in primary nursing the recipient of this service or product is directly or indirectly the patient.

The first skill required of the middle manager is planning and organizing. This involves the analysis of data so that pertinent facts may be extracted or problems identified. Based on this foundation, a workable, flexible plan focused at goal attainment may be developed.

Specific skills required in planning and organizing include:

1. Setting objectives,
2. Outlining the project,
3. Assigning individuals the work,
4. Determining the method of project accomplishment, and
5. Determining what resources/equipment are required.

Each of these skills must complement the others to create a cohesive project and attain the desired outcome.

The skills of planning and organizing can be exemplified within the managerial role of primary nursing. For example, one of the essential components of primary nursing is continuity of patient–nurse assignments. Therefore, in planning and organizing staffing patterns, this component must be retained. The middle manager must analyze the total number of staff available for patient care needs, allocation of that staff, and alternatives for staffing crises.

Another planning and organizing skill required is that of delegation. Delegation is the assignment of a task and/or the giving away of responsibility and authority. In primary nursing the middle manager delegates responsibility for direct patient care management to the primary nurse. The middle manager supports this delegated role through a resource-consultative function. Such delegation is clearly defined as an expectation when the middle manager consults with the primary nurse regarding patient problems and progress, asks appropriate questions of the direct care giver, and serves as a clinical resource.

Appropriate allocation of staff is crucial to enhance primary nursing and, therefore, is an additional organizational skill required by the middle manager. This involves interviewing staff candidates, planning assignments, and evaluating and adjusting personnel to meet patient care needs.

Each new potential professional nurse interviewed provides an opportunity to strengthen the mode of patient care delivery utilized within a nursing service. Therefore, the initial interview must be aimed at assessing the strengths and weaknesses of the applicant in relationship to primary nursing. It is the responsibility of the middle manager within primary nursing to develop interviewing skills that enable him or her to make valid personnel selections.

Figure 5.1, "Interview Selection Process," illustrates the conceptualization of the interview process. During the interview, the middle manager and the applicant must both obtain and give information related to primary nursing. The middle manager's dialogue must include (1) the implementation of the concept

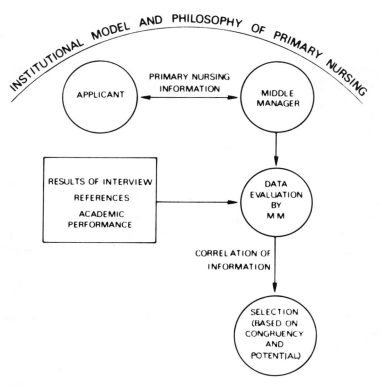

**FIGURE 5.1.**    Interview selection process.

within the agency, (2) the specific skills required and methods available for development, and (3) expectations.

The middle manager must solicit the applicant's knowledge of the concept of primary nursing, experience in concept application, level of clinical skills, and the support of the philosophy of this mode of patient care delivery. These data may be obtained through direct questioning techniques, discussion, or patient care simulations. Table 5.1, "The Interview Guide for Obtaining Information from Potential Primary Nurse Applicants," outlines the process that may be used to obtain these data.

**TABLE 5.1.**
## Interview Guide for Obtaining Information from Potential Primary Nurse Applicants

| Information Desired | Communication Technique Questions such as: |
| --- | --- |
| Knowledge of Concept of Primary Nursing<br>　A. Essential Components of Delivery Systems<br>　B. Role of Professional Nurse | 1. Based on your understanding, what is primary nursing?<br>2. What are the most important aspects of primary nursing?<br>3. As a primary nurse, what is your role?<br>4. Within this role, what are your responsibilities?<br>5. What activities would fulfill these responsibilities?<br>6. How does primary nursing differ from team nursing? |
| Experience in Concept Application | 1. In your basic nursing program, what clinical experience did you have in a primary nursing setting?<br>2. In what modes of patient care delivery have you worked?<br>3. If you practiced in a primary nurse setting, describe your role.<br>4. Based on your experience in the primary nurse model, what do you see as the strengths and weaknesses in the system? |
| Level of Clinical Skills | 1. Based upon the responsibilities and related activities of the primary nurse, what skills are crucial to the role?<br>2. Rate yourself on the following, or give examples:<br>　a. Verbal communication (with peers, M.D.s, paraprofessionals, or other disciplines)<br>　b. Technical skills |

*(continued)*

c. Utilization of the nursing process
d. Written communication
  1. Nursing care planning
  2. Documentation
e. Decision making
f. Utilization of resources
g. Utilization of principles of physiology and psychology
h. Patient advocacy role

---

Following the initial interview, the data obtained must be validated and evaluated by the middle manager. Sources of validation and additional information supportive of primary nursing are not restricted to the immediate verbal interview, but may also be obtained through references and academic evaluations. Although the applicant may demonstrate deficits related to primary nursing on interview, the middle manager must assess whether these may be remedied through an educational program available within the service or whether they are fundamentally incompatible with the concept.

After all the data are obtained and reviewed, the middle manager must correlate this information with the institutional model and philosophy of primary nursing, and the selection process commences. Selection depends upon the congruency between the requirements of the institution and the skills and philosophy of the applicant.

When an applicant is selected for employment within the primary nursing setting, planning and organizing the assignment of the professional nurse to the appropriate unit is part of the middle manager's role. Many staffing methodologies currently use patient classification systems as the sole guide for staffing requirements. Although this system is valid in assessing patients' needs for nursing care, additional factors must be considered when assigning primary nurses. These factors include the skill of the nurse and the support systems available on the particular unit.

One of the keys to successful primary nurse implementation is the appropriate assignment of the primary nurse. Therefore careful consideration must be given to this sensitive task. Orientation to the concept of primary nursing or to the particular ward is not the direct responsibility of the middle manager. However, he serves as a resource and facilitator to the planning and organizing of the orientation process. This becomes even more crucial in staffing crises, when planning alternatives may have to be utilized.

In planning and organizing, the first step of the management process, daily staff allocation requires particular middle managerial attention. The middle manager within primary nursing must establish criteria upon which reassignment or "floating" of staff maintains the integrity of the system. This can be maintained only when "floating" is based upon the needs of the patient and the skills of the nurse. For example, given two primary nurses who are available for reassignment, the one whose primary patient requires goal accomplishment during that shift remains on the original unit.

During a crisis, if reassignment becomes essential, partial shifts or several hours should be used as alternatives rather than full tours. The middle manager needs skill in obtaining data regarding patient goals and assessing the urgencies of meeting these goals. If a primary nurse is not floated because of priority patient need, the middle manager is responsible for follow-up on goal attainment.

Another example of managerial planning and organizing is the utilization of deliberate goal-directed activity, commonly referred to as management by objectives (MBOs). The middle manager in a primary nurse setting must ask herself the following questions to formulate service objectives:

1. Is the objective statement related to and consistent with the nursing service philosophy?
2. Is the objective statement constructed properly?
   a. Contains an action verb

    b. Contains a single key result
    c. Establishes a target date
    d. Establishes an estimated cost
3. Is it measurable and verifiable?
4. Is the objective a realistic and attainable one that still represents a significant challenge to the manager and his staff?
5. Can it be readily understood by those who must implement it?
6. Will the result justify the expenditure of time and resources to achieve it?
7. Can the accountability for final results be clearly established?

MBOs congruent with the basic concepts of primary nursing facilitate its growth. It is the middle manager's role to determine that MBOs are developed in an organized, prioritized manner. During the implementation phase of primary nursing, MBOs that move from the simple basic goals to sophisticated objectives solidify the models.

Once the planning and organizing is accomplished, the middle manager in primary nursing must direct and motivate personnel toward goal attainment as defined in the MBOs. Directing is the "doing" phase of the middle managerial role. This includes such activities as:

1. Assuring adequate materials, time supplies, and staff,
2. Establishing and communicating expectations, standards, and roles for individual personnel involved,
3. Coordinating activities,
4. Integrating viewpoints,
5. Maintaining relationships,
6. Controlling costs,
7. Documenting progress, and
8. Building and maintaining a positive, productive, and stimulating environment.

Motivation of staff for purposes of this discussion is defined as the removal of obstacles to accomplish preestablished goals. Since much has been written about this concept, refer to the references cited in this chapter for further in-depth reading on the topic.

In primary nursing the middle manager has the opportunity to remove multiple obstacles in the implementation process. One clinical example of the middle manager directing/motivating involves the development of a method to insure continuity of patient care between shifts. A method of communicating patient data must be established, and a commonly used technique is walking rounds. This allows for communication between the primary nurse, secondary nurse, and patients. Walking rounds are the process of verbally communicating and usually assessing the patient at the bedside.

Common obstacles in implementing this method of between shift reports include:

1. Time required,
2. Cost,
3. Maintenance of patient,
4. Skill deficits of nurses in communicating and assessing in this manner,
5. Ability of professional staff to involve the patient and family,
6. Interruptions of staff, and
7. Ward coverage during rounds.

To accomplish establishment of walking rounds on a given unit, both the first-line and middle manager must remove the obstacles listed above, thereby insuring the opportunity for the staff to be motivated to reach this goal.

Directing the implementation of walking rounds includes:

1. Stating explicit expectations,
2. Allocating time for walking rounds,

3. Teaching skills and procedures through demonstration,
4. Allowing uninterrupted time to accomplish rounds, with specific coverage for other patients,
5. Obtaining feedback from staff, in order to improve the procedure and maintain relationships between the primary and secondary nurse, and
6. Establishing procedures for communicating data.

Utilizing such techniques can promote the accomplishment of a specific MBO such as establishing walking rounds.

The final phase of the managerial process which must be used in the middle manager's role is controlling. Controlling involves the evaluation of outcomes based upon preestablished criteria and taking corrective action as indicated.

Patient care outcomes are the focus of controlling activities in primary nursing and are effected by both personnel and environmental conditions and supplies. Therefore, in primary nursing the middle manager must evaluate the effects of both these components singularly and in combination. For example, if a primary nurse demonstrates deficits in written documentation of patient care activities after an extensive educational program and repeated counseling by the head nurse, the middle manager must then evaluate these behaviors based on total patient outcomes, and take corrective actions. These may include removal from the role of primary nurse, withholding an advancement, transferring to another area, or dismissal. Another example of middle managerial control focuses on the investigation of high incidences of infection in a given area. Such items as poor handwashing facilities, faulty sterile equipment, or patient placement are items that may account for a high rate of nosocomial infections. Corrective actions include procurement of supplies and facilities to implement infection control measures.

An example of patient care outcomes that involve the interplay between personnel and environment is the absence of specific equipment needed in isolation, indicating that primary nurses are not following preestablished procedures. In this example, the middle manager, in conjunction with the head nurse, must correct both the supply and technique problem before positive patient outcomes can be achieved. The utilization of the management process involves organizing and planning, motivating, directing, and controlling. This process is used in all patient care modalities, but within primary nursing the middle manager focuses on activities related to patient outcomes.

## COMMUNICATION EFFECTIVENESS

Effective communication skills are of prime importance and are integrated into every component of the management process. The art of transmitting information is similar within every patient care delivery system; however, in primary nursing selected aspects require emphasis. A review of some basic principles of effective communication include the following:

1. Communication within an organization is a planned activity and a process from which all other functions derive.
2. Communication is found in all aspects of the management process.
3. Communication may be upward, downward, or horizontal from the sender.
4. Ineffective communication is not cost effective.
5. The perceiver of the message interprets its meaning.
6. Communication may be verbal or nonverbal.
7. One communicates in all interactions.
8. Repetition of the message improves communication.

9. A mechanism for feedback enhances communication effectiveness.
10. Communication is a message sent and received. (Metzer, 1978, pp. 68–69).

Prior to communicating a message, the middle manager needs to determine whether he desires to exercise managerial power and authority, or influence. This decision will determine the technique by which the message is communicated. For example, if the middle manager gives a directive, the communication style should denote that no choices are available to the perceiver. On the other hand, if advice is the purpose of the interaction, then the middle manager offers the receiver a choice. In primary nursing, the middle manager must select what is appropriate for directives versus that which he wishes to influence.

Another aspect of communication that requires emphasis in primary nursing may be labeled the "jargon." This occurs in both verbal and nonverbal communication.

Nonverbal communications that are important to review for primary nursing jargon include many familiar tools used in all systems. The terminology used in policies, job descriptions, minutes, and memos must refer to the primary nurse and be consistent with the basic elements of the concept. Evaluations must refer to the nurse in her primary role. An example of a nonverbal communication tool that must be eliminated within a primary nursing service are such familiar tools as Team I and Team II temperature boards. Traditional assignment sheets do not reinforce the concept of primary nursing nor communicate it to other health care service. This could be replaced by the utilization of a primary nursing color-coded bulletin board. The objective of this tool is to visualize the following:

1. Assignment of the patient to his or her nurse on admission.

2. Daily assignment of primary patients and secondary patients.
3. Assignments of nonprofessionals to accountable primary nurses.

Other uses of this bulletin board include in-service assignments, visibility of the quality of patient care planning and documentation, and medical staff assignments. The evaluation of the planning and documentation by the individual primary nurses are shown via a colored dot system which designates quality. This board is illustrated in *Nursing 79*, October, page 55.

The middle manager's role in implementing such communication tools is to:

1. Assist the head nurse in their development,
2. Obtain needed supplies,
3. Facilitate implementation, and
4. Serve as a role model.

The middle manager can act as a role model by consistently utilizing such a nonverbal primary nursing communication tool.

The verbal terminology should also be consistent with the concept. In daily interchange, the middle manager must be cognitively aware of the verbal phraseology she uses to convey messages to personnel on the unit and within management. One must avoid the use of such terms as "team leader" and "team member," and convert to the utilization of terms such as "primary nurse" and "secondary nurse."

The message of primary nursing—the importance of the primary nurse in patient care outcomes—must be conveyed in conferences between middle managers and first-line personnel. For example, if during a head nurse conference falls were discussed, it is important for middle management to directly request data from the primary nurse rather than intermediaries such as the head nurse. Therefore, the question addressed to the head nurse group would be, "Based upon your primary nurses' assessments, what are the factors which might attribute to the high incidence of patient falls in the last month?"

The communication network within the system of primary nursing is rather unorthodox. In traditional systems, the network follows the organizational chart in a hierarchical manner. In primary nursing, the source of patient-related data becomes the primary nurse, be it the staff or head nurse. For example, when the supervisor must obtain reports and patient classification data, it is the primary nurse's role to categorize her patients and determine what data is important to communicate. One written tool to facilitate this pattern of communication between the primary nurse and the supervisor is the "supervisor's worksheet." On this worksheet, the names of the patients are listed, as well as previous shift's classification. When the primary nurse is on duty, she notes pertinent data and the current classification of the patient. For primary nurses not on duty, this becomes a responsibility for either the secondary nurse or the professional with overall ward responsibility. Figure 5.2 illustrates this worksheet.

Supervisory communication with other disciplines and departments is direct as in traditional systems. However, the middle manager must be aware that the primary nurse in her autonomous role also has the prerogative of this type of communication with other health care services. The middle manager must convey to the primary nurse and first-line manager what her expectations are in relationship to interdepartmental primary nurse communication. Another example of direct primary nurse communication is with the patient's family. Communication related to patient's status and outcomes should be direct between the primary nurse and family, with the middle manager used as a resource to facilitate that interaction.

Another important communication area is related to interpersonal relationships. Metzer (1978, p. 60) states that middle managers tend to waste energies and resources because they

| Bed No. | Patient Classification (Day Shift) | Name | Data | Patient Classification (P.M. Shift) | Comments |
|---|---|---|---|---|---|
| 1 | II | John Jones | B/P stable | II | |
| 2 | I | Mary Mack | irregular pulse confused | I | See me, S. Jones, P.N. |
| | | | | | |

**FIGURE 5.2.** Supervisors worksheet.

concentrate on the form of communication rather than the substance. Substance can be obtained only through the skill of listening and allowing the primary nurse and first-line managers to verbally problem solve independently.

Through interpersonal skills such as listening, the supervisor can convey the message that the primary nurse can have the freedom to practice professionally. Included in this message is the permission to be creative, and to select nontraditional methods to meet patient needs. Middle managers will become more adept at the "art of listening" in primary nurse and first-line managerial interactions if the following principles are observed:

1. Use selective and judicious silence.
2. Ask open-ended questions rather than give answers.
3. Listen for feelings.
4. Be aware of your own biases.

If the middle manager retains jargon found in other delivery systems, she is relaying a confusing message and condoning retention of prior delivery systems.

The middle manager's role in communication is to gain the cooperation of nursing staff to facilitate primary patient care. In primary nursing, this requires skillful communication between the patient care giver or the primary nurse and the supervisory staff.

## APPLICATION OF TEACHING AND LEARNING PRINCIPLES

In primary nursing, the middle manager must be adept at the application of teaching and learning principles and in the identification of those elements that must be taught. The basic principles of teaching and learning as defined by Pohl (1968, pp. 6–45) are consistent in the middle managerial role in all patient care delivery systems. These principles include:

# I. Principles of Learning

A. Readiness is a prerequisite for learning.
B. Learning requires goal setting.
C. Learning requires motivation.
D. New learning must be based on previous knowledge and experience.
E. Learning is affected by emotions.
F. Learners are individuals.
G. Repetition strengthens learning.
H. Satisfaction reinforces learning.
I. Information that applies to daily work is learned more readily than irrelevant information.
J. Learning requires active involvement.

# II. Principles of Teaching

A. Teaching requires motivation.
B. Good teacher–learner rapport is important in teaching.
C. Teaching requires effective communication.
D. Objectives serve as guides in planning and evaluating teaching.
E. Teacher must know materials to be taught.
F. Teaching skill can be acquired through practice and observation.
G. Teacher must be flexible.
H. Sameness causes boredom.
I. Control of the environment is essential.
J. Evaluation is an integral part of teaching.

When implementing primary nursing, it is important for the middle manager to assess the staff's desire to improve in the quality of patient care delivered. This forms the basis for their readiness and motivation for change. The middle manager must assess the skills and abilities staff possess and, based on this foundation, build additional competencies. Realistic goals must then be established which are achievable within a reasonable amount of time, allowing for individual variance.

Staff satisfaction will be greater if active involvement in the change process is encouraged and the emotional climate is positive. The middle manager must teach those elements of primary nursing that are relevant to the daily delivery of quality care. This facilitates reinforcement and relevancy.

Employing the principle that "control of the environment is essential," it is important for the middle manager to recognize that all environments have the potential for teaching and learning, and appropriate opportunities must be capitalized upon. Judicious use of both traditional educational environments and clinical interactions will allow the middle manager opportunities to discuss, consult, role model, and reinforce appropriate behaviors.

A second function of the middle manager is to determine instructional content. This requires knowledge of primary nursing. Primary nursing can be divided into the implementation and sustaining phases. The implementation phase can then be subdivided into two subdivisions: that of teaching rudimentary skills within the concept, and second, synthesis of the professional role. During the initial phase of implementation, the middle manager must focus on: (1) cognitive knowledge of primary nursing, (2) patient care assessment, (3) care planning, (4) documentation, (5) verbal reporting, (6) assignment tools, and (7) decentralized communication techniques.

The assessing, planning, documenting, and reporting skills are usually taught through the head nurse and, therefore, it is the direct responsibility of the middle manager to develop these skills in the head nurse.

Two additional areas of concentration in phase I focus on the head nurse developing the skills of time management and decentralization of authority. Time management skills include the planning of hours to facilitate continuity of patient care. For example, the head nurse must learn to correlate primary nurse vacations and days off with a corresponding decrease in patient caseload.

Another management skill the head nurse must develop is allocating time for patient care conferences. Primary patient care conferences do not require the time commitment of other modalities because the plan of care has already been developed (Mayer and Bailey, 1979). The middle manager can demonstrate that this mode of communication is most effectively instituted at a ten-minute session during change of shift.

Decentralization of authority is a crucial concept and requires breaking very old and traditional habits. In primary nursing, the authority in patient care is the primary nurse, and the head nurse must learn the consultant's role. To facilitate this learning, the middle manager must teach the head nurse the socratic method of problem solving. The effective head nurse leads the primary nurse through programmed instruction and solicits from that individual suitable alternative solutions. The most effective communication technique is the questioning method. This helps develop creative problem solvers.

In the synthesis of the professional role, the major outcome desired is an independent practitioner, be it the head or primary nurse. To accomplish this goal, the middle manager must be flexible in her role. Initially, the middle manager is the teacher, demonstrator, evaluator, and consultant. As the head or primary nurse begins to demonstrate initial competencies, the middle manager weans the professional nurse and begins to encourage assertiveness, advocacy, autonomy, authority, and accountability. This weaning process is extremely difficult since it implies chronic role change for the middle manager and great diversity in interactions among individuals in a service.

When primary nursing has been implemented, the sustaining phase ensues, in which the middle manager focuses on the development of long-term behavior. Definitions of these 5 A's have been adapted from Watts and O'Leary (1980) and are as follows:

1. Advocacy—the process by which one pleads the case of another
2. Autonomy—the commitment to self-direction or initiation of independent action
3. Authority—the right to utilize power or control to influence or command others
4. Accountability—acceptance of responsibility for the ultimate results of action taken
5. Assertiveness—indication of appropriate behavior or feeling

During this phase the middle manager must continue to promote the sophistication of already learned skills and knowledge through constant evaluation and reinforcement. Table 5.2, "Summary of Instructional Content for Middle Managers," summarizes the instructional content in the phases of implementation of primary nursing.

In some health care facilities, this initial educational process is a dual responsibility of both management and education. However, the program must be coordinated and be a major focus of the entire service. Therefore, the middle manager must be a skilled teacher and evaluator of learning.

## UTILIZATION OF CHANGE PRINCIPLES

The decision to implement primary nursing within a nursing service requires expertise in the utilization of the change process. The principles of change remain constant within all types of delivery systems; however, the success of the implementation of primary nursing is dependent upon skilled usage of this process. Therefore, a review of the change process is germane.

Change within an organization may be defined as any alteration within the environment. Change may be planned or unplanned. Planned change derives from a deliberate effort to alter

## TABLE 5.2.
## Summary of Instructional Content for Middle Managers

| Implementation | Target Group | Content Areas |
|---|---|---|
| Phase I | Primary Nurse and Head Nurse | Concept knowledge<br>Assessment<br>Planning<br>Documentation<br>Reporting<br>Communication<br>Tool utilization |
| | Head Nurse | Use of basic skills in management<br>  Time allocations<br>  Decentralized authority<br>  Weaning |
| Phase II | Primary Nurse and Head Nurse | Advocacy<br>Autonomy<br>Authority<br>Accountability<br>Assertiveness |
| Sustaining | Primary Nurse and Head Nurse | Evaluation of skill utilization<br>Sophistication of skills |

some condition which has been stimulated by either internal or external forces. Unplanned change is a response to some stimuli in an effort to reestablish organizational equilibrium.

Change tends to upset the status quo of individuals within an organization psychologically, socially, and economically. Therefore, it is crucial that the middle manager be cognizant of why change is resisted and of methods to overcome this obstacle.

Individuals within an organization converting to primary nursing may resist change because of both psychological and social factors. An example is the fear of failure in demonstrating essential skills required of the primary nurse. Second, a change may be caused in the social structure of the unit, and the individual may be required to reestablish relationships within a setting that may be threatening. For example, within the team system, the team leader's position is one of interdependency. This changes dramatically in primary nursing because of the autonomous nature of the primary nurse role. Language symbols that provided security in one system now are replaced with the "jargon" of primary nursing, and relearning and restructuring is required.

Psychosocial resistance also occurs when a change is not clearly understood and expectations are vague. This creates psychological uncertainty and requires a major investment of energy in the attempt to comply and cope with the change.

Economically, resistance to change stems from fear of losing one's job, inconvenience, and uncertainty of the future.

According to Metzer (1978, pp. 57–58), techniques utilized in overcoming resistance to change include:

1. Acknowledge that resistance is a symptom of some underlying causal factors.
2. Allow release of feelings.
3. Allow groups' input in the identification of problems and making of decisions.
4. Promote a positive work milieu.
5. Utilize constructive, positive, two-way communication inclusive of
   a. Reason for change
   b. Plan for change
   c. Projected effect on personnel.

The change process that is currently in vogue has been described by Kurt Lewin. This process involves unfreezing, changing, and refreezing.

The aim of unfreezing is to motivate and prepare personnel for the change desired. This is accomplished by making the personnel aware of the need for change. An example of unfreezing related to the introduction of primary nursing is to ask the nurse to identify elements of quality nursing care that are valued. A next step is to correlate these valued elements with several modes of patient care delivery. The patient care system which allows the delivery of the valued elements of care promotes identification of the need for change. Once individuals see the need for change, the middle manager assists in the actual planning and implementing of the desired changed behavior.

The last step of this change process is refreezing or the process by which the newly acquired behavior is solidified as recurring behavior. An environment must be created which reinforces the changed behavior so it can become internalized. After the change has occurred, middle management must reinforce, comment, and complement, to help refreeze this new behavior. This is an element of the managerial process called the phase of control.

A positive approach to the introduction of change is a skill the middle manager must develop and use. Table 5.3, "The Positive Change Process," describes the steps for implementation of positive/productive change.

The utilization of the change process being implemented in a positive fashion within primary nursing is exemplified in the conversion of the assignment of primary nurses to patients. Specifically, this involves the middle manager interacting with the head nurse in the implementation process.

When the modular system, based on geographic location of beds, is changed to assignment based upon patients' needs and nurses' skills, the need for change is identified. In the modular assignment system, new orientees are unable to demonstrate the clinical competencies required to deliver care to all patients in a module. In addition, nurses' skills frequently do not meet pa-

## TABLE 5.3.
### The Positive Change Process*

| Steps for Positive Change | Description of Steps |
|---|---|
| 1. Identification | Staff recognizes that the problem exists within their milieu |
| 2. Reassurance | Alleviations of fears associated with change |
| 3. Communication | Utilization of effective means of conveying change |
| 4. Participation | The process of obtaining input and feedback related to changes |
| 5. Mutual Interest | Correlation of proposed change to value system |
| 6. Follow-through | The process of detecting weaknesses and strengths of the change |

*Adapted from Stuvert, 1959.

tients' needs. Finally, the modular system means equalization of patient caseload and not necessarily workload.

Reassurance is given to the nursing personnel that primary nurses can be relieved on a daily basis when the stresses and strains of a difficult patient create undue burden. This is a concern when movement from a modular system is suggested. In addition, nurses are assured that through appropriate assignments and knowledge of the needs and interventions appropriate for their patients, the time required in nongeographical assignments will be compensated.

In communicating to the staff, the middle manager and the head nurse explain the process and rationale for the change in detail. At this time, they invite participation in the development of tools to be used in communicating assignments, patient assessments, and the mechanics of making assignments. The implementation of the change invites mutual interest through participation and personal investment in the project.

The last function of the middle manager and the head nurse in this change is to provide follow-through by means of evaluation on all shifts and long-term revisions to facilitate assignment bases upon nurses' skills and patients' needs.

The smooth transition to primary nursing is facilitated by the sophisticated utilization of the change process. Although many managers have had basic change theory in the educational setting, effective clinical application is not consistently practiced. Therefore, special attention must focus on this middle managerial skill.

## IMPLEMENTATION

The process of implementing primary nursing takes a long-term commitment by both management and staff. It includes sequential planning, delegation, coordination of activities, communication, and follow-up.

Primary nursing is best implemented on the basis of two stages. Phase I is basic skill development, previously discussed, and is aimed at converting from one delivery system to another. In Phase I, the middle manager serves as a mentor and consultant to the head nurse in setting the specific objectives that will improve those staff nurse skills required in primary nursing. Examples of the target group, specific objectives, and selected criteria which are appropriate for Phase I include those listed in Table 5.4, "Phase I: Implementation of Primary Nursing."

Behavioral changes must be demonstrated by those individuals identified in the target group in order to accomplish each objective in Phase I. The criteria outlines methods by which the objectives might be accomplished and evaluated.

Table 5.5, "Phase II: Implementation of Primary Nursing," explains information similar to that found in Table 5.4 for the second phase of implementation. The development of an independent practitioner is a goal of Phase II; therefore, the middle

## TABLE 5.4.
## Phase I: Implementation of Primary Nursing

| Target Group | Objective | Examples of Selected Criteria |
|---|---|---|
| Head Nurse | Assigns primary patients to primary nurses based upon skills of the nurse and needs of the patient. | 1. Patients are assigned nongeographically. 2. Nurse competencies are congruent with patient needs. |
| Head Nurse | Assigns primary patients to the primary nurse when on duty. | 1. Patient have consistent nurse assignment at least 70 percent of the time. |
| Head Nurse/ Staff Nurse | Identifies the primary nurse as the principle care giver for her primary patients. | 1. The name of the primary nurse will be visible to patient, nursing staff, other disciplines, and support services. |
| Primary Nurse | Plans patient care based upon 24-hour patient needs. | 1. Writes nursing care plan within 24 hours of admission. 2. Signs ordered nursing interventions. 3. Reviews goals and objectives for patient care. 4. Adapts nursing care plan to patient's changing needs. |
| Primary Nurse | Documents patient's progress toward goal achievement. | 1. Charts when on duty. 2. Correlates documentation to patient's problems. 3. Charts status of patient for inter-ward transfer. 4. Discharge plans and summaries are clearly detailed in chart. |

*(continued)*

| Target Group | Objective | Examples of Selected Criteria |
|---|---|---|
| Primary Nurse/ Head Nurse | Demonstrates decentralized communication. | 1. Information requests regarding patients will be referred to primary nurse.<br>2. Primary nurse communicates directly to other disciplines and to secondary nurse. |
| Primary Nurse | Plans for patient discharge. | 1. Nursing care plan reflects patient discharge needs inclusive of supplies, placement, and support systems.<br>2. Primary nurse writes appropriate, complete referrals on primary patients.<br>3. Primary nurse institutes a discharge program and documents patient knowledge level. |
| Primary Nurse | Reports patient data and plan of care to other health care givers. | 1. Directly communicates to off shifts and other disciplines.<br>2. Gives report on own primary patients. |
| Primary Nurse | Assesses patient's physical, and psychosocial needs. | 1. Completes admission data base within 24 hours of admission.<br>2. Documents admission on progress notes. |
| Primary Nurse | Conducts primary patient conference aimed at communicating plan of care. | 1. Presents plan of care to staff on own primary patients. |

## TABLE 5.5.
## Phase II: Implementation of Primary Nursing

| Target Group | Objective | Examples of Selected Criteria |
|---|---|---|
| Primary Nurse | Demonstrates authority in patient assessments, communication, and evaluation of the plan of care. | 1. Correlates overt observations with physiological and psychosocial theory.<br>2. Demonstrates decentralized communication skills to relay data associated with patient assessment.<br>3. Takes appropriate action to alter the nursing care plan based upon patient data. |
| Primary Nurse | Utilizes skills of assertiveness in interactions with health care providers and support services. | 1. Verbalizes nursing orders using, "I, the primary nurse . . .". |
| Primary Nurse | Demonstrates patient advocacy in planned nursing interventions and communications with nursing staff and other disciplines. | 1. Incorporates the patient as a collaborator in discharge planning. |
| Primary Nurse | Demonstrates autonomous nursing actions based upon sound application of theory and prioritization | 1. Independently establishes and implements actions to meet patient needs and goals.<br>2. Makes nursing judgments based upon patient priorities. |

(*continued*)

| Primary Nurse | Demonstrates accountability in the planning, delivery, and evaluation of primary patient care. | 1. Maintains 24-hour responsibility of patient care inclusive of:<br>a. Up-to-date communication via nursing care plan<br>b. Verbal direction to secondary nurses<br>c. Documentation of patient's progress toward goal achievement and problem resolution. |
| --- | --- | --- |

manager's role is one of facilitating this independence. This is accomplished through a process of step-wise "weaning" which occurs at both the staff and head nurse levels. The middle manager becomes a teacher/mentor to the head nurse in planning individualized "weaning" programs for each primary nurse. In addition, the middle manager must reinforce head nurse behaviors that productively elicit desired staff nurse independence.

In turn, as the staff nurse role changes into one of a primary nurse, the head nurse role evolves into one of staff developer and resource person. The middle manager supports this role evolution and adapts accordingly.

Rewards of this system are different from those in traditional modalities, and, therefore, the middle manager must be supportive to the head nurse. For example, in traditional models the head nurse frequently communicates directly with the physician. If this is viewed as rewarding to the head nurse, decentralization of communication to primary nurse authority and direct communication may create a "void" within the head nurse. Other rewards such as demonstrated primary nurse growth and patient satisfaction must be seen by the head nurse as positive job accomplishments during the complex implementation process.

# EVALUATION

The term *evaluation* denotes the process of making a judgment related to the usefulness or value of something. In this process, a comparison is established between an object or program and a yardstick or standard of acceptability. There are generally five standards used in evaluation, and they are as follows:

1. Historical Standard       a measure of an object before and after

2. Normative Standard      comparison of one group against another

3. Absolute Standard       100 percent achievement

4. Theoretical Standard     expected results if everything went right, based on best evidence from previous research

5. Negotiated Standard     may want 100 percent but will settle for a lesser degree

Evaluation within primary nursing must occur to document the results of implementation. The middle manager may select any one of the five types of standards of evaluation previously described for this process. Though it does not matter which one of the standards is utilized, objectives and criteria must be established prior to the evaluation. Samples of criteria are found in Tables 5.4 and 5.5.

The absolute and negotiated standard may be used at any stage of Phase I and Phase II to evaluate the implementation of a given set of objectives. For example, in Table 5.4 an absolute standard is employed and measurement involves assessing assignment patterns, and numerically tabulating adherence. Another objective states, "Assigns primary patient to primary nurse when on duty," and that this should occur 100 percent of the time. Therefore, an objective states, "The primary nurse will conduct primary care conferences aimed at communicating the plan of care" which can be judged under a negotiated standard since 100 percent compliance is not crucial. It may be decided that only 50 to 75 percent of patients require a conference of this type.

The historical standard may be employed by the middle manager to depict baseline data prior to the implementation of a given change. Evaluation following the change is then geared toward achievement of the goal. For example, prior to efforts to implement primary nursing on a ward, data may be collected to describe the current status of patient assignments, documentation, charting, and so on. Following planned change, data will demonstrate growth and development in these areas.

If one ward is compared to another, a normative standard is in use. An example would be testing the effectiveness of an assignment board on different wards. A comparison could be made of one ward to another.

An example of a theoretical standard of evaluation could be utilized in determining cost effectiveness of primary nursing versus other modalities utilizing Gwen Marram's study as the theoretical base (Marram et al., 1976).

The middle manager must have a working knowledge of the various types of evaluation and be able to select the most appropriate standard.

## INTERACTION WITH ORGANIZED LABOR

Change has occurred within the nursing profession and has permeated the world of relationships between management and staff personnel. With the evolution of professional nurse unionization, the manager within a primary nursing setting must be cognizant of the impact and ramifications of organized labor.

Maintenance of a constructive and productive work environment is dependent upon the value that first-line and middle management personnel place upon cohesive relationships and actions aimed at service goal accomplishments.

The middle manager's role in a primary nursing unionized setting evolves around two major categories of activities: (1) the role in negotiating a contract, and (2) the role in implementation of the contract. Each activity will be discussed in separate subheadings.

## Negotiating the Contract

Prior to the labor and management team going to the negotiation table, the middle manager must be accountable for analyzing those aspects of the proposed contract that have implications for primary nursing. For example, areas to consider include (1) hours and shifts, (2) overtime, (3) absence from duty, and (4) assignments and reassignments. These areas should be analyzed for congruency with the concept of comprehensive, continuous, coordinated, individualized, and total patient care.

Hours and shifts must be reviewed to give the primary nurse the flexibility to respond to primary patients' individualized needs. This is illustrated in patients who have not been taught and are discharged without prior notice. The primary nurse may need the flexibility to return to duty that evening to prepare the patient adequately for discharge the following morning. Flexible, approved shifts may be needed to implement primary nursing.

The criteria and procedure for overtime must also allow flexibility for the primary nurse. Consideration for overtime should be based upon the needs of specific primary patients rather than the commonly used standard of equal distribution of hours. When equitable distribution becomes the major criterion, the focus of the system shifts from a patient- to a staff/hospital-centered philosophy. This is incongruent with primary nursing. The needs of the patients must be of primary importance in granting absence from duty. This is true if it be a one-day workshop or a week's annual vacation. The union contract usually addresses the procedure for requesting and approving these types of leaves of absence. The ramification for the middle manager is to focus on meeting the needs of the primary patients in the absence of the primary nurse. For short-term absences this may be accomplished through the use of a secondary nurse. For long-term absences, a plan must be available so that continuity and coordinated care can be maintained. Prior to planned vacation, patient assignment should decrease so that there is an attrition of caseload. For extended vacations, primary patients may have to be reassigned.

When a middle manager is considering reassignment of a primary nurse to another unit, consideration of current primary patients must be assessed. Following assessment, the middle manager's actions through the head nurse may include reassigning the patient to another primary nurse, delaying the transfer until there is closure of the primary nurse–patient relationship, or allowing flexibility for the transferred primary nurse to return to the original unit to meet specific, predetermined patient needs.

Previous chapters have discussed the short-term reassignment of primary nurses.

## Implementing the Contract

The mode of patient care delivery within a nursing service does not dictate the principles the middle manager must follow in contract implementation. Once the contract is agreed upon by management and labor, it is too late to rectify incongruencies between the agreement and primary nursing.

The role of the middle manager in contract implementation focuses in four major areas:

1. Teaching first-line managers the content of the contract,
2. Controlling adherence to the contract agreement,
3. Identifying incongruencies with primary nursing and assisting the head nurse with constructive methods of adaptation, and
4. Promoting resolutions of potential formal grievances at the lowest organizational level possible.

Through the period of negotiation and following finalization, head nurses must furnish input and review the final product. This is most simply accomplished through comparison between old and new contracts, with identification of the areas of major change.

The middle manager acts as the controller in assuring contract adherence at all levels. She should be available for consultation when questions arise at the head nurse level. In addition, routine checks on critical issues should be made to identify and avoid inadvertent infractions.

During the implementation phase of a new contract, areas of incongruencies with primary nursing should be identified and noted. This should be followed by collective problem solving so there will be the least amount of negative impact on the primary nursing model, patients, and nurses.

The final major role of the middle manager in relationship to union contracts that will be discussed here is the avoidance of formal grievances and the resolution at the informal level. This is done primarily by employing open and skilled communication between the members of the bargaining unit and first-line managers. It is the middle manager's role to identify deficits in head nurse communication skills and to direct concentrated efforts toward improvements.

## MIDDLE MANAGER'S JOB DESCRIPTION

In the patient-focused delivery modality of primary nursing, the middle manager's role is diverse and aimed at the delivery of comprehensive, coordinated, continuous, individualized total patient care. In the previous sections, the middle managerial skills requiring development have been discussed.

Within a nursing service employing primary nursing, it is important to have job descriptions congruent with the concept. Therefore, the middle manager's role description is very important. Usually, the job description of the staff nurse has undergone significant changes congruent with primary nursing. These changes were primarily in the areas of communication, accountability, authority, and patient care planning. In contrast, the middle manager's role has remained the same for all patient care modalities. Herein lies an irony that creates role conflict between the staff primary nurse and the middle manager.

The following middle manager's job description, Table 5.6, "Job Description: Middle Manager," is one example that reflects the concept and the skills previously discussed.

# TABLE 5.6.
## Job Description: Middle Manager

*I. Role of Supervisor (Middle Manager)*

The Supervisor of Nursing Service is accountable for patient care through managerial, supervisory, and evaluative skills utilized in interactions with nursing and other personnel on specified units. The minimum preparation should be a baccalaureate degree and two years of successful clinical practice in related areas. The Supervisor will promote and maintain his or her role and responsibilities through skilled utilization of the nursing, management, and change processes, application of teaching/learning principles and cognitive/theoretical nursing knowledge, and demonstration of effective communication techniques. The Supervisor is responsible to the Director of Nursing Service for patient care management.

*II. Functions and Responsibilities*

The Supervisor is accountable for four major areas of jurisdiction (patient care, education, research, and administration).

A. Patient Care
1. Assesses nursing care plans, implements needed changes, and evaluates results of actions consistent with primary nursing.
2. Evaluates the quality of patient care, utilizing the auditing process and multidisciplinary and nursing rounds.
3. Communicates with patients by seeking out and listening to their opinions concerning care received.
4. Acts as a clinical resource.
5. Maintains effective communications related to patient care with other services.
6. Participates in primary nursing conferences.

*(continued)*

B. Research
1. Improves nursing care and administrative functions through utilization of relevant research.
2. Participates in appropriate research projects.

C. Education
1. Improves the performance and clinical skills of primary nursing personnel through staff development programs.
2. Establishes congruency between nursing policies and procedures, and primary nursing.
3. Maintains and promotes current knowledge related to nursing practice.
4. Collaborates in the planning, implementing, and evaluating of staff development programs.
5. Assists the Head Nurse in development of skills required for his or her role within primary nursing.

D. Administration
1. Maintains staffing congruent with the concept of primary nursing.
   a. Provides effective staffing on a 24-hour basis.
   b. Projects future staffing needs.
2. Assesses and makes recommendations for structural changes, equipment, and supplies.
3. Recruits Nursing Service personnel.
4. Plans, initiates, and evaluates programs for patient care services within Nursing Service and other disciplines.
5. Formulates objectives for Nursing Service through collaboration with appropriate Nursing Service personnel.
6. Evaluates performance of nursing personnel and provides for their professional development.
7. Formulates policies, procedures, job descriptions for nursing personnel.

# Chapter 6
# The Nursing Clinical Coordinator

Many nursing services that have implemented primary nursing have abolished the traditional supervisory role. The new role that has developed in primary nursing settings is the nursing clinical coordinator. It is a combination of the traditional head nurse and the clinical specialist role. This individual is usually a clinical nurse specialist in a related area who has had administrative experience. She is a clinical expert and serves both as the role model and consultant in patient care, and administratively performs such duties as evaluation of personnel, construction/implementation of unit objectives, and facilitation of organizational communication.

The traditional supervisor is one step away from the patient because of hierarchical organizational patterns. The nursing clinical coordinator is next to the primary nurse, in close proximity to the patient, both clinically and administratively. This is more congruent with the philosophy of primary nursing than the traditional supervisory position. Figure 6.1, "Traditional Organizational Chart," illustrates the traditional layering of an organization. Figure 6.2, "Organizational Chart Within Primary Nursing," demonstrates the organizational structure with the Nursing Clinical Coordinator.

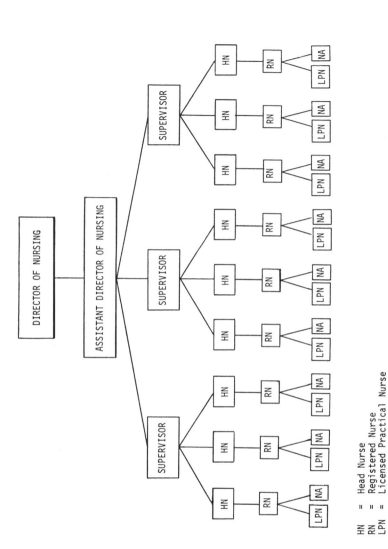

HN = Head Nurse
RN = Registered Nurse
LPN = Licensed Practical Nurse
NA = Nursing Assistant

**FIGURE 6.1.** Traditional organization chart.

79

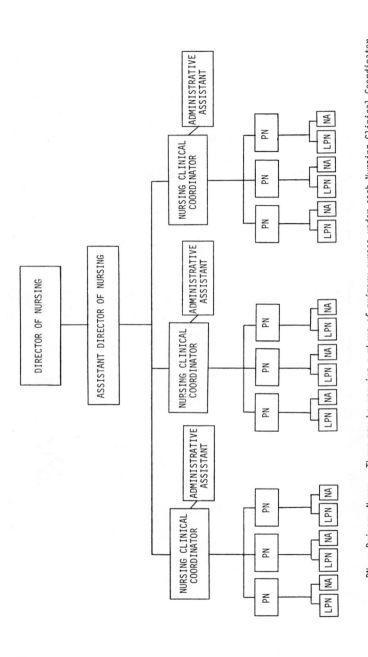

PN = Primary Nurse – There may be varying numbers of primary nurses under each Nursing Clinical Coordinator
LPN = Licensed Practical Nurse
NA = Nursing Assistant

**FIGURE 6.2.** Organizational chart within primary nursing.

As depicted in Figure 6.2, each clinical care coordinator is assigned an administrative assistant to provide support for clerical and routine, administrative work. These tasks include requisition of supplies, requests for repairs, time planning, and so on. Examples of a job description of the nursing clinical coordinator and the administrative assistant, Tables 6.1 and 6.2, respectively, are found at the end of this chapter. The job description of the clinical coordinator is consistant with the skills needed by the middle manager outlined in Chapter 5.

There are many benefits in implementing this system, which utilizes the clinical coordinator in conjunction with primary nursing. First, this system places the expert in patient care at the bedside. With the clinical and administrative roles combined, problems are solved utilizing the "best of both worlds."

Second, nonlayering of the organizational structure has ramifications in the realm of communications and budget. Removal of one administrative layer and combining two roles allows for more direct communication between top and first-line management. Control from one level to the second level can be more consistent. Patient needs, therefore, are communicated more directly, and the old game of "telephone" can be eliminated. With improved communication and decreased chance of error, costs may be reduced. In addition, removing one category of personnel decreases staffing costs at high administrative positions. The funds secured from this savings could therefore be utilized for salaries of administrative assistants or additional primary nurses.

Third, placing the clinical expert at the bedside improves patient care decisions, thereby reducing "trial and error" decision making. In a day of accelerating health care costs, it would behoove nursing directors to consider these organizational factors in implementing the primary nursing model.

Another benefit of this combined role is the credibility established when the supervisor is the most competent practitioner. Administrative and clinical directives and judgments are most often accepted by primary nurses when given by managerial

# TABLE 6.1
## Position Description: Nursing Clinical Coordinator

*I. Role*

The Nursing Clinical Coordinator (NCC) is a registered professional nurse responsible to the Director of Nursing Service or delegated assistant. Competencies required include demonstrated clinical and educational expertise.

*II. Functions*

The NCC is accountable for:

A. Patient Care Delivery
   1. Implementing and maintaining the concept of primary nursing on the unit in order to deliver individualized, comprehensive, coordinated, and continuous total patient care.
   2. Guiding the primary/professional nurse in the use of the nursing process, and in the development and utilization of the nursing care plan for all patients.
   3. Assisting the primary nurse in the utilization of other disciplines for consultation, planning, assistance, and advice in meeting patients' needs.
   4. Assuring that primary nurses are accountable for documenting care given, family/patient teaching, and discharge planning for primary patients.
   5. Delivering direct patient care for purposes of identifying and meeting patient needs, maintaining clinical expertise, and serving as a role model to primary nurses.
   6. Implementing changes in patient care as indicated by Quality Assurance Programs and current research findings.

*(continued)*

7. Evaluating the quality of individual patient care based on the current concepts of patient care management and standards.

8. Serving as a patient advocate.

9. Directing, evaluating, and maintaining a safe environment for the promotion of patient care delivery.

B. Unit Management

1. Planning a ward management program based upon an ongoing system of written objectives consistent with the philosophy and objectives of the Service.

2. Participating on Nursing Service committees.

3. Evaluating and documenting staff performance, counseling as needed, and making recommendations for promotions.

4. Conducting regular staff meetings for the communication of pertinent information and participation of staff.

5. Appraising planned time schedules for nursing personnel, using principles of time planning, hospital policies and guidelines, and contract agreements.

6. Delegating non-nursing administrative functions to appropriate staff.

7. Developing and maintaining operational policies, procedures, and guidelines that enable the unit to function in an organized and efficient manner.

8. Facilitating written and verbal communication related to the nursing unit.

C. Clinical Inquiry

1. Initiating and participating in nursing studies and research projects.

2. Identifying relevant research and findings, and using when appropriate.

3. Coordinating nursing studies conducted on the unit.

(continued)

D. Staff Development

1. Providing and evaluating an individualized orientation program in conjunction with nursing education for all unit employees.
2. Providing opportunities for staff development through patient conferences, in-service programs, bedside teaching, staff projects and assignments, and serving as a resource person.
3. Implementing the principles and resources that promote teaching and learning.
4. Promoting a motivational climate that encourages staff growth, development, and morale.
5. Organizing a unit in-service program that promotes standards of nursing care and current trends in nursing practice and communicates policies and procedures.
6. Providing individual learning experiences for nursing personnel based upon identified needs.
7. Supporting and participating in the promotion of learning experiences for nursing students, as well as students from other health disciplines.
8. Teaching in centralized educational programs.

personnel who also possess skilled clinical competencies. This enhances role modeling, communications, and professional commitment throughout a staff and has implications for promoting staff development and retention.

One of the major deterrents to adopting this system is tradition, both institutional and educational. Tradition has dictated that a nurse be either a practitioner or an administrator, and the combination is relatively rare. In addition, hospitals may have a strong supervisory staff that is unwilling to adapt to a new system and role. Educationally, programs do not prepare students for the combined role, serving to further complicate the recruitment process.

Another problem involves developing the role and securing the position of an administrative assistant. In these times of budgetary restraints, the addition of another nonclinical person may be difficult for the hospital administration to endorse. However, this position is crucial if the nursing clinical coordinator is to have time to meet the expectations required by the new role.

In summary, a nursing clinical coordinator with an administrative assistant is more congruent with the philosophy of primary nursing than are other traditional supervisory positions. Efforts to implement these roles must be supported by data and concrete budgetary figures.

# TABLE 6.2
## Position Description: Administrative Assistant

*I. Role*

The Administrative Assistant (AA) provides administrative/managerial support to the Nursing Clinical Coordinator (NCC). The AA will be delegated responsibilities for non-nursing duties. The AA is accountable to the NCC and is expected to organize and establish priorities in a self-directed manner.

*II. Functions*

The AA is accountable for:

A. Secretarial correspondence, dictation, minutes, etc.
B. Collecting and collating data and maintaining preidentified reports, surveys, and requests for information.
C. Maintaining an administrative calendar and/or file related to personnel matters.
D. Maintaining current procedure and policy files.
E. Requesting procurement of new equipment and maintaining current equipment.
F. Planning and reviewing time and vacation schedules following preestablished guidelines.
G. Assisting the NCC in procurement of staffing in emergency situations.
H. Collecting data concerning patient classification to assist in decision making.
I. Securing clinical resources such as literature, audiovisuals, etc.

# Chapter 7
# Expectations and Rewards

Expectations of the middle manager in primary nursing are numerous. The middle manager can expect the health care organization to demand that patients receive quality care, that patients and employees be satisfied in the setting, and that this be accomplished in a cost-effective manner. The middle manager is expected to evaluate, managerially control, and have an effective follow-up program when deficits in these areas are noted.

The middle manager must also have institutional and professional goals and expectations. For example, the middle manager must be knowledgeable about the concept of primary nursing and principles of management and be able to synthesize these into one congruent whole. In addition, to fulfill the role of consultant, the middle manager must have a "bag full of alternatives" to promote the implementation and maintenance of primary nursing models within financial restraints.

Such high personal and institutional expectations are not without associated frustrations. In the process of the role change previously described, three frustrations arise: those within the manager, those arising from within the organization, and those inherent in the profession of nursing.

One common personal frustration for the middle manager is impatience with the change process. Examples of areas that move slowly in primary nursing include the evolution of the head nurse's and middle manager's roles, and the staff nurse's development of primary nurse skills, such as autonomy, authority, assertiveness, accountability, and advocacy. These are long-term developmental processes that require not only solid planning and foresight but patience and good humor. Other examples of areas that move slowly are policy changes, staffing ratios, equipment acquisitions, and attitudes.

Other frustrations that arise are loneliness within the middle manager's role and lack of peer support. When there are several middle managers within a service, each manager evolves into the middle managerial role at a different pace. This creates incongruencies within the same role, thereby isolating individuals and decreasing support among peers. However, this has the potential to create internal competitiveness among middle managers, which can be healthy when limited but when unidentified and uncontrolled can be fairly destructive.

As primary and head nurses' competencies increase, their roles expand and become more diverse. This affects the middle manager's role. Initially, this creates a feeling of incompetence, bewilderment, and role confusion in the middle manager, until she can develop and create the new role.

External frustrations revolve around the organization and the nursing profession. All organizations have traditions. These may include the traditional organizational structure with the physician in the predominant role or with nurse–patient relationships. One of the most difficult traditions common in health care facilities is that of inertia, maintaining the status quo, or the tradition of not changing.

Examples of common organizationally related frustrations for the middle manager in primary nursing include coping with the bureaucratic, hierarchical structure, lack of adequate support systems, and only passive support during the implementation process of primary nursing.

A hierarchical structure without flexibility makes role change extremely difficult. Unless the organizational structure can allow the decentralization of patient care authority, implementation of primary nursing will be extremely difficult. Vacillation between centralization and decentralization yields role confusion for both the primary nurse and the middle manager. The middle manager may be caught between patient care and administrative demands.

Support systems are crucial to the successful implementation and continuous growth of primary nursing. Primary nurses must have the freedom to provide nursing services to their primary patients instead of housekeeping, clerical, pharmaceutical, and escort patient services. These departments must have the person power to supplement unit needs. The dilemma occurs when nursing is forced to assume these tasks, thus cheating primary patients of nurses' professional care.

The administrative decision to implement primary nursing must be reinforced both verbally and by action. Frustration occurs when the middle manager receives only verbal support coupled with inaction or counter action. For example, administratively it is imperative that an R.N. staff ratio be maintained that supports the delivery system practiced. Research indicates a minimum R.N. to nonprofessional ratio is 60:40. When nursing is cut short due to staff cutbacks, resignations, and high turnover, the middle manager experiences the disintegration of an "unfrozen" primary nursing model and a high frustration level.

The final middle managerial frustration that is extremely common is related to the nursing profession and associated educational preparation. Traditionally, the educational process prepares the nurse manager to function in a hierarchical, centralized type of organizational structure. Therefore, this basic preparation is incongruent with primary nursing and requires relearning.

The rewards of the middle manager within primary nursing evolve from a traditionally administrative role to one that includes components of clinical practice, staff development, and research. With this expansion of the role, the middle manager's function and responsibilities in patient care outcomes become more clearly delineated.

Specifically, middle managerial rewards are documented

through quality assurance programs. For example, the quality of patient care delivery can be measured through retrospective and concurrent audits, incidence reports, and nosocomial infection rates. Second, quality of care may be measured indirectly through patient and family satisfaction studies. When positive data are retrieved from these sources, the middle manager receives reinforcement that the system is functioning well.

Another area of satisfaction is related to staff development. As the primary nurse and head nurse begin to demonstrate growth in their primary nursing roles and associated skills, there is actualization of patient-centered care. This in itself is an area that provides the middle manager with rewards and has the potential for increasing staff satisfaction. A satisfied practitioner who can visualize self or professional growth leads to a stable staff with improved retention. Once staff achieves basic primary nursing competencies, it is easy to move forward to more complex skills rather than repeatedly orienting a new staff to fundamental skills.

A direct source of middle managerial rewards comes from top management and is related to those mentioned above. As documented data support quality of patient care and staff retention increases, top managerial goals are realized. These are explicitly identified in yearly middle manager's evaluations and indirectly in annual reports and/or verbal feedback. Finally, the middle manager may experience personal satisfaction in a role that combines all aspects of nursing and is not restricted to the administrative component.

The middle manager must be cognizant of the expectations, frustrations, and multiple rewards that are an outgrowth of the transition from traditional modes of patient care delivery to primary nursing. Through identification of these elements, the middle manager is better prepared for the inherent stress found in the change process.

# Part II
# Bridging the Gap

---

## BEING A MIDDLE MANAGER IS NOT QUITE THE SAME AS BECOMING ONE

The development of the middle manager's role in primary nursing requires many adaptations. These include personal, professional, and organizational changes. What are the problems that impede the transition and adaptations? What support systems are available to the middle manager to facilitate these changes? What is the role of the educational institution? How can nursing services facilitate the change institutionally?

If nurses believe in patient-centered care, why has there been such a problem in role transition? Once problems have been identified, it is prudent to identify alternative solutions. The following chapters attempt to do this.

# Chapter 8
# Current Problems

Middle managerial deficits in primary nursing stem from problems that originate in three major areas of concentration:

1. Educational preparation of the professional nurse,
2. Qualifications of personnel, and
3. Institutional programs.

In order to suggest alternative solutions, an identification of specific problems in each area is essential.

## EDUCATIONAL PREPARATION

The backbone of any type of nursing practice is the educational preparation and competencies of the individual practitioner. Middle managers are prepared in both undergraduate and graduate programs, and knowledge deficits in this process are reflected in application and performance on the job.

Traditionally, undergraduate education focuses on the nurse–patient interrelationship rather than the systems in which that relationship develops. To develop practitioners within primary nursing, the theory of the concept must be studied. Therefore, the first problem identified in educational preparation is that the practitioner does not have the basic concept of various delivery systems, including primary nursing. That is, the graduate does not set professional goals in terms of the development of primary nursing skills.

This problem is seen when didactic instruction lacks introduction to the primary nursing delivery systems and offers only minimal practice in laboratory and clinical settings. Practice within clinical settings utilizing primary nursing provides the opportunities for students to see and apply the concept. When information about primary nursing has been presented in the classroom and reinforced clinically, synthesis of learning occurs. But when faculty lack skills and experience in primary nursing, they cannot guide students in this modality or serve as a role model.

Undergraduate education is not intended to prepare students specifically for the middle manager's role in primary nursing, but it should provide both the theoretical and experiential basis of introduction to the concept. When this framework is lacking at this level, it is difficult to fill the gap.

Another educational area that creates problems in primary nursing is related to change and leadership theory competencies. The concept of primary nursing as practiced and implemented today requires skilled utilization of these theories. For example, most institutions need to "change" to primary nursing from a more traditional patient care modality. If change theory is not used appropriately with effective leadership, primary nursing usually does not succeed.

Traditionally in undergraduate programs the nursing process is taught as a theoretical framework for professional practice. This provides the basis for practice and patient care interventions.

A third problem area is that the management of patient care is frequently a neglected topic. Minimal correlations are made between the use of the nursing process in the organization and the delivery system in which that care takes place. A beginning understanding of the management process is essential to effectively deliver optimum care within a health care facility. In the undergraduate program, the care of more than one primary patient requires beginning management skills. The integration of the nursing management process needs to occur when the movement from a single to multiple patient assignment occurs.

Current problems related to primary nursing in undergraduate education are usually correlated with the lack of theoretical basic knowledge and clinical experience in the concept. In associate or diploma nursing programs, terminal objectives usually do not focus on leadership/management theory; therefore, as we discussed earlier, difficulties in utilizing these graduates without supplemental educational preparation in the managerial role creates a reliance on "learning via osmosis."

In graduate education, students are encouraged to select specific tracts focusing on either clinical practice, education, administration, or research. These specialty areas create the establishment of a role specific to only one area of nursing. It is unreasonable to think that middle managers in primary nursing can administrate units and staff, practicing in this modality, unless they have additional skills in education and clinical practice. This lack of integration creates a serious problem within the middle manager's role. The longer graduate programs pursue isolated divisions, the longer professional practice will be deprived of potential resources (Moritz, 1979).

When a student does select an administrative tract, emphasis is usually placed on the top managerial position, that of the Director of Nursing Service. Students usually participate in one-to-one preceptorship with a Director of Nursing and become knowledgeable at this level of decision making. Little emphasis is given to the middle manager's role except as it interfaces with top management. Yet in many instances, attainment of a top management position upon graduation is somewhat unrealistic and advancement to this top level position is often attained through evaluation at the middle manager's level.

Most graduate curricula emphasize leadership and management theory but do not stress the variances and emphasis required in different patient care modalities. Therefore, the graduate is under the false assumption that management is management, and the skills required are the same in all systems. Obviously, principles and certain skills are the same, such as planning, organizing, motivating, and controlling; however, such skills as delegation, practice of authority, and some aspects of communication are different. The development of these specific skills is a necessity for the successful middle manager in primary nursing.

Preceptorships at the graduate level frequently are designed with objectives that do not measure any success or failure in the competencies required in the manager's role. Rather, objectives frequently will analyze, dissect, and recreate the role instead of make it operational. Clinical settings have difficulty in redirecting the objectives when previously approved by the educational institution.

As indicated in the undergraduate programs previously discussed, graduate students also lack adequate primary nursing middle manager's role models as preceptors and/or instructors. Coupled with poor theoretical preparation and clinical application, this lack leads to a severe problem. If middle managers are to be administrators of patient care, then educational institutions must provide the opportunity both to examine the appropriate theory and to apply the theoretical concepts clinically.

## QUALIFICATIONS OF PERSONNEL

A large problem exists in the qualifications of individuals currently expected to fulfill the role of the middle manager in primary nursing. Nursing has created a "catch as catch can" situation and supported "osmotic learning." This is illustrated in a complete lack of a conceptualization of the role as indicated in the literature, and in practice. Analysis of current middle manager job descriptions usually reveal a void in skills required to perform this job successfully in a primary nursing setting. These problems may be due to limited educationally sponsored clinical practice, poor role models, or lack of experimentation in creating an effective role. Nursing in middle management many times prefers to make tradition "king."

Currently, resources are usually targeted to another population, the head and primary nurse. Therefore, upon analysis of the present situation, resources are sadly lacking in the establishment of this role. This creates a gap of qualified personnel at a very important point in the organizational chart. The head and primary nurses may be forced to revert back to traditional practices if the middle manager cannot operate in a primary nursing system.

## INSTITUTIONAL PROGRAMS

Staff development programs within health care institutions are most frequently targeted at the staff nurse level. Very few programs are established for middle and top management. The philosophy underlying this void in middle management programming is "a manager is a manager is a manager." This attitude fosters simplicity in problem solving. It is indeed correct that managerial principles remain the same at all levels whereas the complexity of application increases. Therefore, staff development programs must be targeted at levels of management rather than management as a whole.

Institutionally, if the middle manager's role is to be implemented, goals must be set and time allocated for this purpose. It is a dangerous assumption that the middle manager is too busy to acquire the skills required to implement the role change. In total, such an attitude within a service can destroy the entire primary nursing system.

The successful evolution of the role of the middle manager within primary nursing is dependent upon three major factors: educational preparation, qualifications of personnel, and institutional programs. The consequences of gaps among these three create deficits that must be resolved for successful implementation of the role.

# Chapter 9
# Bridging the Gap Educationally

The outcomes and consequences of a chasm existing between education and service were discussed in the previous chapter. It behooves progressive nursing leaders with the common goal of the delivery of quality care through primary nursing to come to grips with these problems. This requires careful analysis and creative problem solving for both service and education. This chapter will propose some alternatives for bridging the gap educationally.

## UNDERGRADUATE PROGRAMS

Terminal behaviors of basic nursing graduates should be congruent with the concept of primary nursing to provide a baseline for future managerial positions. Therefore, the first step in bridging the gap educationally is to analyze terminal program objectives. This should be followed by appropriate revisions of terminal and course objectives, as well as curricular content related to primary nursing. Some suggested examples of terminal and related course objectives are seen in Table 9.1, "Terminal and Course Objectives for Basic Nursing Programs Related to Primary Nursing."

**TABLE 9.1.**

**Terminal and Course Objectives for Basic Nursing Programs Related to Primary Nursing**

| *Terminal Objectives* | *Course/Clinical Objectives* |
|---|---|
| The student will be able to: | The student will be able to: |
| 1. Utilize the nursing process in a variety of patient care delivery modalities. | 1. Describe the following types of patient care delivery systems:<br>  a. functional<br>  b. team<br>  c. case<br>  d. modular<br>  e. primary<br>2. Compare/contrast the following elements of five delivery systems:<br>  a. major focus<br>  b. accountability<br>  c. authority lines<br>  d. communication patterns<br>  e. bases of personnel assignment<br>  f. patient care planning<br>3. Define the nursing process.<br>4. Discuss the utilization of the nursing process within the different delivery systems.<br>5. Clinically demonstrate the utilization of the nursing process in selected delivery modalities. |
| 2. Demonstrate the primary nurse role clinically. | 1. Describe the role of the primary nurse in relationship to patient care.<br>2. Based upon a selected preceptorship, analyze the role of the primary nurse. |

*(continued)*

3. Integrate into practice multiple leadership processes.

3. Demonstrate clinically the role of the primary nurse for selected patients.
4. Analyze personal implementation of the primary nurse role for identification of strengths and weaknesses.
5. Implement a plan to increase primary nurse skills.
1. Describe the change and management processes utilized in the leadership role.
2. Compare/contrast the change and management processes as utilized within selected patient delivery systems.
3. Implement clinically beginning levels of the change and management processes within the primary nursing framework.

---

The objectives in Table 9.1 can be adapted for both associate and baccalaureate programs dependent upon the philosophy of the school. However, it must be emphasized that both terminal and course objectives should address the concept of primary nursing to provide the basic framework and a suitable reference for the middle manager in this patient care modality.

A second focus which aids in bridging the gap educationally evolves from selection of appropriate faculty, along with a statement of their expectations. It is difficult to teach the essence of primary nursing without having basic knowledge of the concept and personally applying it clinically. Since primary nursing is relatively new, many faculty members have not had the opportunity to practice in such a setting. It is strongly recommended that faculty have the prestated obligation to practice primary nursing clinically prior to teaching it. This can be accomplished by preceptorships within a primary nursing setting or working during academic breaks or sabbatical leaves. Such a faculty program would provide instructors with both theoretical and practical experiences with the concept. In addition, the faculty would then have the opportunity to practice primary nursing role modeling and to analyze the process of being an example in a clinical setting. From personal professional experience in primary nursing, the teacher would find the transfer to student classroom instruction and clinical application more meaningful, realistic, and practical.

## GRADUATE PROGRAMS

Graduate nursing education furnishes the opportunity for the student to develop in depth various concepts related to management. The principles of management remain constant within curricula; however, specifics of application may vary according to the framework of practice.

In the previous chapter, the problem of tracting in graduate programs was discussed as it relates to primary nursing and the middle manager. To bridge the gap at this level, graduate program terminal objectives must focus on the development of clinical, administrative, educational, and research competencies. Although specific professional choices must occur, single tracting should be avoided early in the graduate educational process because both primary nursing and management principles can be related to all aspects of practice.

Some examples of terminal objectives related to primary nursing and the middle manager are seen in Table 9.2, "Graduate Terminal and Course Objectives Related to Primary Nursing." These objectives are intended to serve as general guidelines.

The objectives stated in Table 9.2 would be applicable to any of the study tracts commonly pursued in graduate study and should be included in the curriculum. If a student were in a tract emphasizing clinical practice, heavy emphasis would be placed on terminal objectives 1, 2, and 5. If, however, the graduate student were in the administrative tract, terminal objectives 1

## TABLE 9.2.
### Graduate Terminal and Course Objectives Related to Primary Nursing

| Terminal Objectives | Course/Clinical Objectives |
|---|---|
| The student will be able to: | The student will be able to: |
| 1. Integrate into a leadership primary nursing role competencies of clinical practice and principles of management and staff development. | 1. Describe a leadership role within primary nursing. 2. Analyze the primary nursing leadership role for application of specified clinical competencies, principles of management, and staff development. 3. Demonstrate clinical competence, principles of leadership, and staff development in a managerial role within a primary nursing delivery system. |
| 2. Analyze the role of the middle manager in primary nursing utilizing scientific principles and a research methodology. | 1. Identify a researchable problem associated with the role of the primary nurse/middle manager. 2. Review the literature related to the problem. 3. Develop a methodology. 4. Implement the preestablished methodology. 5. Analyze data. 6. Summarize data with conclusions and recommendations. |
| 3. Develop an organizational structure supportive of the concept of primary nursing. | 1. Identify methods of organizing a nursing service suitable for primary nursing. 2. Analyze/compare an organizational structure for appropriateness to primary nursing. |

(continued)

| | |
|---|---|
| 4. Develop a plan to implement primary nursing, considering elements of clinical practice, administration, education, and research. | 3. Develop an organizational structure compatible with the concept of primary nursing.<br>1. Identify elements of primary nursing related to clinical practice, administration, education, and research.<br>2. Develop objectives and action plans for implementation of primary nursing including the elements identified above.<br>3. Discuss modalities of implementation incorporating principles of change. |
| 5. Demonstrate skills required of the middle manager in a primary nursing setting. | 1. Identify skills needed by the middle manager.<br>2. Develop a plan for implementation of skills.<br>3. Implement skills.<br>4. Evaluate impact. |

through 5 would be of equal importance. Finally, an educational tract would emphasize terminal objectives 1, 2, 4, and 5.

The suggestions proposed for undergraduate faculty are also true for graduate faculty. However, an additional element essential for graduate faculty is the actual practical experience within the primary nursing leadership role. This is necessary because it requires a skilled, experienced faculty to teach a potential leader the skills required to develop subordinates.

Since the implementation of primary nursing is still relatively in its infancy, graduate faculty must participate in research related to the concept at all levels. Doing so would improve faculty ability to develop new and innovative methods of implementation and roles, as well as to evaluate the outcomes of patient care. This may be one of the most essential contributions graduate faculties can make to primary nursing.

Bridging the gap educationally involves curriculum changes in both undergraduate and graduate education, plus securing and maintaining qualified faculty adept at teaching the concept. This chapter has given specific suggestions that can be modified and adapted to a wide variety of institutions.

# Chapter 10
# Bridging the Gap Institutionally

Creative problem solving implemented by nursing leaders within a health care facility can bridge the gap institutionally. It is in the health care institution that the application of knowledge learned in the educational setting is demonstrated behaviorally and clinically. Therefore, in conjunction with a knowledge base, the environment in which application occurs and grows is of equal importance. To implement primary nursing successfully, a thorough analysis of this environment is needed. This must be followed by astute planning, thorough implementation, and ongoing evaluation.

One of the first tasks in analyzing the environment for primary nursing is to determine the types of personnel composing middle management. Staff may be categorized based upon their educational backgrounds and their previous clinical experience or expertise. Educationally, the middle manager may be a product of a traditional program or an innovative one such as the one detailed in the previous chapter. Staff categorization must be based upon clinical and managerial experience, expertise, and previous assignments. These three items may be classified as a positive or negative factor. For example, the experience of a nursing supervisor with longevity within a functional nursing service would be more negative than if equal practice had been in a more innovative patient care modality. Figure 10.1, "Middle Managerial Staff Configuration," represents this concept. Based upon results of the analysis of the middle managerial staff, several configurations of characteristics emerge. Some of the variations are as follows: Individuals who require:

1. Theoretical knowledge
    a. Principles of leadership/management
    b. Principles of primary nursing
2. Practical clinical middle managerial experience within primary nursing.

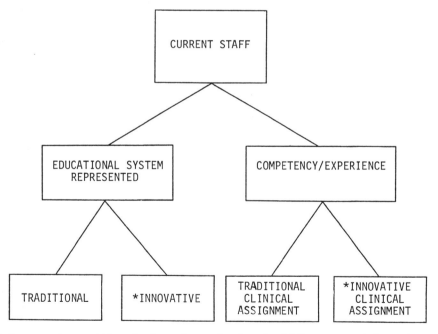

\* Represents positive factors in analysis of middle managerial staff

**FIGURE 10.1.**    Middle managerial staff configuration.

In response to the different needs, it becomes crucial that the institution individualize the staff development program aimed at preparing the middle manager for primary nursing. These programs vary in content and scope and are basically focused upon:

1. Theory,
2. Orientation to the role within primary nursing, and
3. Clinical application.

Table 10.1, "Focus of Staff Development Based upon Staff Analysis," outlines the categories of middle managerial staff and the suggested focus of the staff development program.

Individuals from traditional educational and experience backgrounds should have a program aimed at a total relearning. This would include material related to primary nursing theory, role, and clinical application. Individuals representative of an innovative educational program require materials related to role and clinical application. In contrast, the person who has many years of managerial experience in innovative patient care delivery systems would require only an orientation to the primary nursing role. This is true even if they have had traditional educational backgrounds, since demonstrated clinical competence represents the synthesis of knowledge.

Knowledge of leadership/management theory is the first staff development prerequisite. The following pages present a sample of a basic health facility leadership/management course, which is one alternative solution in bridging the gap institutionally. Included are the conceptual framework, the target group, the general course plan, course objectives, and suggested content.

## 1

*Course Title:* Basic Leadership/Management Course in Clinical Setting
*Target Group:* Potential and current managerial staff

**TABLE 10.1.**
**Focus of Staff Development Based upon Staff Analysis**

| Categories of Middle Managerial Staff | Staff Development Focus | | | |
|---|---|---|---|---|
| | Theory: | | Orientation to Role in | |
| | Leadership/Management | Primary Nursing | Primary Nursing | Clinical Application |
| Educational Background | | | | |
| Traditional | X | X | X | X |
| Innovative | | | X | X |
| Competency/Experience | | | | |
| Traditional clinical assignments | X | X | X | X |
| Innovative clinical assignments | | | X | |

*Conceptual Framework:*  It is suggested that at the basic course level, the framework be built upon the correlation between the nursing and managerial processes.

*Course Objectives:*  At the completion of the course, the participant will be able to:

1. Describe the relationship between the nursing and management processes.
2. Given specific examples, identify the components and application of:
   a. Leadership theory
   b. Change principles
3. Discuss organizational structure in relationship to philosophy, objectives, managerial methodology, and modalities of patient care.
4. Describe the managerial role related to patient care, staff development, and unit management.

| *Suggested Course Content: Related Course Objective* | *Suggested Course Content Areas* |
| --- | --- |
| 1 | Nursing process |
|  | Management process |
| 2 | Change theory |
|  | Leadership theory |
| 3 | Philosophy and objectives |
|  | Organizational structure |
|  | Methods of management |
|  | Modalities of patient care |
| 4 | Quality assurance programs |
|  | Nursing standards |
|  | Teaching/learning theory |
|  | Motivational theory |

Employee evaluation
Counseling and disciplining
Delegation
Relationship with organized labor
Time management

The previously described leadership/management course is intended for individuals with very limited knowledge of basic theory. This course can be utilized for first-line managers. We suggest that for middle managers, the development of an intermediate level course be initiated and targeted to this specific group. An example of such a course is outlined below.

## 2

*Course Title:* Intermediate Leadership/Management Course in Clinical Setting
*Target Group:* Middle Managers
*Conceptual Framework:* (Suggestion: The management process)
*Course Objectives:* At the completion of the course the nurse will be able to:

1. Describe the relationship among the following:
   a. the nursing process
   b. the management process
   c. the middle managerial role
2. Describe the philosophy and objectives, the organizational structure, and the relationship of these to the purposes, goals, and role of the middle manager.
3. Describe the role of the middle manager in various patient care modalities.
4. Identify resources that facilitate administrative decisions.
5. Describe skills, resources, and tools related to the middle

manager's administrative, research, educational, and patient care role.

| *Suggested Course Content:* *Related Course Objective* | *Suggested Course Content Areas* |
|---|---|
| 1 | Correlate the nursing process, management process, and job description |
| 2 | Correlate role of middle manager to organizational goals, philosophy, and structure |
| 3 | Role/skills of middle manager in different care modalities |
| 4 | Patient care evaluation systems |
| | Standards of patient care |
| | Policies and procedures |
| 5 | Recruitment |
| | Interviewing |
| | Staffing modalities |
| | Time planning |
| | Personnel policies |
| | Counseling |
| | Disciplinary actions |
| | Equipment |
| | Supplies |
| | Problem resolution through research |
| | Problem resolution through educational means |
| | Career development |

Theoretical content related to primary nursing can be integrated into either of the previous two courses described. In the Basic Course, it could be discussed under Objective 3, "modalities of patient care." In the Intermediate Course, it could be discussed under Objectives 2 and 5.

To introduce primary nursing to the middle manager, an additional course may be developed or integrated into the Intermediate Course. Introduction to primary nursing consists of two components, theory and clinical application. The course described next focuses primarily on theory.

## 3

*Course Title:* Patient Care Delivery via Primary Nursing
*Target Group:* Middle Managers
*Course Objectives:* At the completion of the course the participant will be able to:

1. Describe the primary nursing modality and its crucial elements.
2. Utilize the crucial elements of primary nursing in the conceptualization of a ward/service model.
3. Describe the process of primary nursing implementation.
4. Discuss first- and second-line managerial implementation.
5. Discuss skills required to meet role expectations.
6. Design an educational program aimed at the development of these skills.

| *Suggested Course Content:* *Related Course Objective* | *Suggested Course Content Areas* |
|---|---|
| 1 | Compare delivery modalities |

|   | Primary nursing crucial elements |
|---|---|
|   | Role of primary nurse |
| 2 | Necessary elements of ward/ service models |
|   | Stages of implementation |
| 3 | Steps of implementation |
|   | Anticipated problems and rewards |
| 4 | Role of head nurse |
|   | Role of middle manager (Chapter 5) |
| 5 | Skills required (Chapter 5) |
| 6 | Educational programs |

When developing an orientation program for middle management in primary nursing, attention must be given to both knowledge and clinical application. Suggested objectives for an orientation program aimed at clinical application would include the following:

1. Describe the historical development of primary nursing within the specific health care facility.
2. Discuss the correlation of the service's philosophy and objectives to the organization chart to primary nursing.
3. Review job descriptions of all nursing service personnel.
4. Review individual ward primary nursing models.
5. Discuss the elements of the educational program aimed at primary nursing skill development.
6. Identify resources available to support primary nursing (e.g., policies, procedures, standards, personnel, support services).
7. Identify the middle managerial role in relationship to primary nurses, head nurse, other supervisors, and top management.

8. Observe middle manager role model in clinical interaction.
9. Demonstrate utilization of the primary nursing middle managerial skills during preceptorship.

Objective 9 is the clinical application of leadership/management theory, the primary nursing concept, and the unique role within the specific health care facility. During a preceptorship, success in role implementation should be measured by preestablished criteria. Examples of the criteria might include the following:

1. Demonstrates decentralized communicaion patterns in ward interactions.
2. Assigns nursing personnel aimed at promotion of continuity of patient care.
3. Consults with primary nurse regarding patient care goals and problems.
4. Utilizes problem solving techniques in staff development.
5. Utilizes resources appropriately.
6. Identifies practices that are congruent and incongruent with primary nursing.
7. Identifies primary nursing skill deficits and seeks resolution in a creative manner.
8. Promotes primary nurse patient care conferences.
9. Demonstrates clinical expertise in the resolution of selected patient care problems.
10. Identifies alternative resources available to primary nursing in resolution of patient problems and goal attainment.

In the annual performance evaluations of the middle manager in primary nursing, emphasis must be placed on the evaluation of these same competencies. Itemizing skills well done serves as a reinforcement for the continuation of these behaviors. In contrast, identifying skill deficits facilitates goal setting and statement of expectations. This promotes growth within the middle manager.

In the process of bridging the gap between education and the health care institution, the unification model may be of value. The unification model combines practice and teaching in the single role of teacher and practitioner, thereby uniting the expert in the science of nursing and the art of practice. This helps to close the gaps previously discussed related to primary nursing, because such a combined role joins the elements of theory and clinical application.

It is unrealistic to assume that all health care facilities have the educational resources to fully implement the educational program previousy described. Such nursing services must look to other viable alternatives. One of the first and most easily accomplished tasks may be the provision of literature focusing on primary nursing, its implementation, and the roles of component personnel. This can be done by the purchase of selected books and periodicals. (See Bibliography at the end of this text.)

The use of consultants in the field of primary nursing is strongly encouraged. A consultant can be used to develop the instructional program and to teach available nursing service personnel methods of implementation and role change. In many instances sources of consultants may include colleges, hospitals that have already implemented primary nursing, and national experts in primary nursing or authors of appropriate literature.

In summary, this chapter has discussed the role of the institution in the development of primary nursing middle managers. This role is not learned through "osmosis," but requires astute, well-planned programs in the nursing service.

# Chapter 11
# Exploration:
# Future Directions

Change invades every aspect of our lives, including our "workaday world and professional careers." This invasion includes health care systems in general, nursing, and its complementary delivery systems and involved personnel. In previous chapters, we have discussed the historical and current perspectives of primary nursing and the middle manager. If our concerted efforts stop at this point, one becomes shortsighted and general myopia pervades. Under such static conditions, neither nursing nor professional personnel can be sensitive and visionary in responding to changing patient needs. A third perspective of equal importance is that of the future. It is important to identify that which may affect health care systems and nursing, and therefore have an impact upon a delivery system such as primary nursing.

It is beyond the scope of this book to discuss all future trends; therefore, the authors have selected those which they feel may have a direct impact on primary nursing and the middle manager. These trends can be divided into the following categories of change:

1. Population
2. Disease patterns
3. Professional nursing
4. Evaluative techniques

## POPULATION

In the future, population trends and changes will affect the entire health care industry. The client population will be older, with divisions of the "young, old" and "old, old." Health care services for these individuals will vary with greater emphasis on long-term care centers outside of the acute care hospital. With this kind of a shift within the populace, coordination among the hospital and the long-term facility, as well as the related services of each, becomes of paramount importance. Ambulatory care facilities will also be affected, delivering health care services to a larger, older population. Hospitalized patients will be admitted for brief periods for diagnostic studies or simple surgical procedures. This is in contrast to the hospitalized patient who is critically ill, requiring sophisticated, complex interventions.

Within this multitude of health care settings, serving a more geriatric population, coordination of efforts and continuity of services aimed at meeting the individualized total client's health needs becomes crucial. This may become the major focus of the primary nurse of the future.

Relevant characteristics of this population that have impact on health care demands include such items as: (1) fixed incomes, (2) higher level of education, (3) transient/mobile living patterns, and (4) decreased impact of the nuclear family. Such characteristics have an impact on health care needs of the individual and demand sensitivity within the system.

A second population trend that has impact upon the primary nurse and middle manager is the increased geriatric population in relationship to a decreased work force. This is demonstrated in a decreased number of available working professional nurses and a decreased enrollment in nursing programs. These factors lead to a younger, less experienced nurse in a middle managerial position. As previously discussed, the middle managerial role within primary nursing is very complex and requires a large variety of professional skills. Therefore, a dichotomy exists. At a time when patient health care needs have increased, the availability of "seasoned" professionals has decreased. In addition, the increased educational requirements of the middle manager tend to favor the younger nurse, who may have achieved educational credentials but lacks clinical experience.

Such population trends create a tremendous burden on the system and the client. Therefore, delivery systems that reduce the stress and address these factors will evolve into the dominant practice. We think that the concept underlying primary nursing is at the present time the only system that is responsive to such stress reduction.

## DISEASE PATTERNS

As the population changes, so will disease patterns. Disease patterns that will merge in the future include those related to longer life, environmental agents, social adaptations, and viral infections. Future progress in each of these areas is directly related to current research findings. This has impact on nursing, since what is relevant today may become passe tomorrow. Therefore, during the professional life of the nurse, it is crucial that educational focus be geared to these changes and that the associated development of clinical competencies aimed at resolving problems be related to these disease patterns.

## PROFESSIONAL NURSING

As changes have occurred in patient populations and disease patterns, so has there been evolutions within the nursing profession. Some of these futuristic trends will have an impact on primary nursing and the roles inherent in the concept.

Educationally, nursing continues to fight for its own professional identity. This is compounded by the multi-levels of educational tracts available to the aspiring nurse and is reinforced by irrational use of the nurse within the clinical area regardless of her basic educational preparation. This accounts for many of the gaps identified. Internally, the profession seems unable to form a consensus on educational preparation and the role of the nurse.

No doubt, external pressures may force a change of viewpoint. The entry-into-practice issue well may end with the baccalaureate degree as the beginning level of professional nursing. Historically, this evolution has been experienced in other fields following much internal turmoil. An example would be the education profession, which within recent decades required collegiate credentials for beginning level practice. Another factor that will cause the increased educational requirement is the large number of other health professionals emerging, many of whom impinge on the traditional territory of nurses. Since these paraprofessionals usually have baccalaureate degrees, nursing will have to follow suit in the very near future to maintain its present place within the health care system.

In the transition years of the '80s, the combination of the baccalaureate degree requirement and an enrollment reduction in educational programs will create a shortage crisis. This will require close scrutiny into the professional role of the nurse and changes in utilization patterns within the health care facility. For example, the middle manager/supervisory role may become a combined clinical-administrative role such as the one described in a previous chapter. This may demonstrate more effective cost control and may even show greater quality of patient care as an end product.

## EVALUATIVE TECHNIQUES

The nursing profession is built upon the nursing process of assessment, planning, implementation, and evaluation. Future trends will see increased emphasis on evaluation. This may be accomplished both internally and externally. Internal evaluation has been emphasized in recent years through retrospective and concurrent audit techniques. The growth of such programs as the Joint Commission of Accreditation of Hospitals, Private Service Review Organizations, and Health Services Review Organizations are examples of external evaluation. The evaluative process is implemented based upon the standards established by these bodies.

The trend toward clinical nursing research and theory building will also affect the patient care delivery systems. Through research, current practices will be evaluated and new techniques and approaches will be discovered and validated. The future will see an increase in all methods of evaluation because of several factors. These include (1) increased sophistication within the profession resulting from increased education, (2) need to control costs, (3) increased health demands by the public, and (4) government regulatory policies and health care programs.

All of these trends will affect patient care delivery systems within a health care facility and the professional roles within the institution. Primary nursing has the potential to be resilient in the face of these projected changes, and the middle managerial role adaptive to the varied patient, professional, and public demands.

# Bibliography

Alfano, G. J. The Loeb Center for Nursing and Rehabilitation—A professional approach to nursing practice, *The Nursing Clinics of North America*, September 1969, *4*, 487–493.

Anderson, M. Primary nursing in day-by-day practice. *American Journal of Nursing*, May 1976, *76*, 802–805.

Anderson, M., Chase, J., and D'Souza, A. M., et al. *Primary Nursing: A Handbook for Implementation* (2nd ed.). Minneapolis: University of Minnesota Hospitals and Clinics, 1978.

Anderson, M., and Choi, T. Primary nursing in an organizational context. *Journal of Nursing Administration*, March 1980, *X*, 26–31.

Arnsdorf, M. B. Perceptions of primary nursing in a family-centered care setting. *Nursing Administration Quarterly*, Winter 1977, *2*, 97–105.

Bakke, K. Primary nursing: Perceptions of a staff nurse. *American Journal of Nursing, 74*, 1432–1434.

Bartels, D., Good, V., and Lampe, S. The role of the head nurse in primary nursing. *Canadian Nurse*, March 1977, *73*, 26–30.

Berkowitz, N., and Malone, M. Intra-professional conflict. *Nursing Forum*, Winter 1968, *3*, 65–69.

Betz, M., Dickerson, T., and Wyatt, D. Cost and quality: Primary and team nursing compared. *Nursing and Health Care*, October 1980, *1*, 150–156.

Block, D. Evaluation of nursing care in terms of process and outcome. *Nursing Research*, July–August 1975, *24*, 256–263.

Bowar-Ferres, S. Loeb Center and its philosophy of nursing. *American Journal of Nursing*, May 1975, *75*, 810–815.

Brown, B. The autonomous nurse and primary nursing. *Nursing Administration Quarterly*, Fall 1976, *1*, 31–36.

Brown, B. J. (Ed.). Nursing education, Part I—Gaps and voids. *Nursing Administration Quarterly*, Spring, 1979. *3*.

Brown, B., Poulin, M. A. (Ed.). Nursing education, Part II—Preparation of nurse administrators. *Nursing Administration Quarterly,* Summer 1979, *3.*

Byers, H., and Klink, J. *Nursing Clinics of North America,* March 1978, *13,* 120.

Carlson, S., Kaufman, R., and Schwaid, M. An experiment in self-determined patient care. *Nursing Clinics of North America,* September 1969, *4,* 495–507.

Christman, L. Accountability and autonomy are more than rhetoric. *Nurse Educator,* July–August 1978, pp. 3–6.

Christy, T. *Cornerstone for Nursing Education.* New York: Teachers College Press, Teachers College, Columbia University, 1969.

Ciske, K. Accountability: The essence of primary nursing. *American Journal of Nursing,* May 1979, 79, 890–894.

Ciske, K. L. *Implementing Primary Nursing: A Study Guide,* Primary Nursing Development, Publishers, 1979.

Ciske, K. Misconceptions about staffing and patient assignment in primary nursing. *American Journal of Nursing,* August 1974, *74,* 61–68.

Ciske, K. and Mayer, G. (Eds.). Primary nursing. *Nursing Dimensions,* Vol. VII, Winter 1980.

Ciske, K. Primary nursing: An organization that promotes professional practice. *Journal of Nursing Administration,* January–February 1974, *IV,* 28–31.

Ciske, K. Primary nursing: Evaluation. *American Journal of Nursing,* August 1974, *74,* 1436–1438.

Clifford, J. The potential of primary nursing. *Health Care in the 1980's: Who Provides? Who Plans? Who Pays?* New York: National League for Nursing, 1979.

Columbia University, Teachers College, Division of Nursing Education. *Regional Planning for Nursing and Nursing Education.* New York: The Macmillan Co., 1948.

Committee on the Function of Nursing. *A Program for the Nursing Profession.* New York: The Macmillan Co., 1948.

Corn, F., Hahn, M., and Lepper, K. Salvaging primary nursing. *Supervisor Nurse,* May 1977, *8,* 19–25.

Corpuz, T. Primary nursing meets needs, expectations of patients and staff. *Hospitals JAHA,* 1977, *51,* 95–100.

Daeffler, R. J. Outcomes of primary nursing for the patient. *Military Medicine,* March 1977, *142,* 204–208.

Daeffler, R. J. Patients' perception of care under team and primary nursing. *Journal of Nursing Administration,* March–April 1975, pp. 20–26.

Dahlen, A. L. With primary nursing we have it all together. *American Journal of Nursing,* March 1978, 78, 426–448.

Dean, L. The changing from functional to primary nursing. *Nursing Clinics of North America*, 1979, *14*, 357–364.

Dolan, J. *Nursing in Society: A Historical Perspective*. Philadelphia: W. B. Saunders Co., 1978.

Dooley, S., and Hauben, J. From staff nurse to head nurse: A trying transition. *Journal of Nursing Administration*, April 1979, pp. 4–7.

Donabedian, A. Patient care evaluation. *Hospitals JAHA*, April 1970, *44*, 131–136.

Donahue, M. Weiner, E., and Shirk, M. Dreams and realities: A nurse, physician, and administration view primary nursing. *Nursing Clinics of North America*, June 1977, *12*, 247–255.

Drice, A. D. Are you a match for primary nursing? *Nursing Careers*, June 1980, *1*, 1–5.

Durand, M. Everybody's patient is nobody's patient. *Nursing Outlook*, September 1975, *23*, 551.

Eichhorn, M. L., and Frevert, E. Evaluation of a nursing system using a quality of patient care scale. *Journal of Nursing Administration*, October 1979.

Elpern, E. Structural and organizational supports for primary nursing. *Nursing Clinics of North America*, June 1977, *12*, 205–219.

Fairbanks, J. N. Staffing a primary nursing unit. *Nursing Administration Quarterly*, Summer 1977, *1*, 79–85.

Felton, G. Increasing the quality of nursing care by introducing the concept of primary nursing: A model project. *Nursing Research*, February 1975, *24*, 27–32.

Felton, G., Frevert, E., Galligan, K., Niell, M. K., and Williams, L. Pathways to accountability: Implementation of a quality assurance program. *Journal of Nursing Administration*, January 1976, pp. 20–24.

Ferguson, F. Staffing: Critical considerations from the perspective of a nursing administrator. *Nursing Administration Quarterly*, Summer 1977, *4*, 46–49.

Frevert, E., and Galligan, K. Evaluation of nursing care: A primary nursing project—Part II. *Supervisor Nurse*, January 1975, pp. 40–43.

Gaynor, A., and Berry, R. Observations of a staff nurse: An organization analysis. *Journal of Nursing Administration*, May–June 1973, *3*, 45–49.

Hall, L. A center for nursing. *Nursing Outlook*, November 1963, *11*, 805–806.

Hall, L. Another view of nursing care and quality. In Straub, M., and Parker, K. (Eds.). *Continuity of Patient Care: The Role of Nursing*. Washington, D.C.: Catholic University Press, 1966.

Hall, M. How do students learn on a primary nursing care unit? *Nursing Outlook*, June 1977, *25*, 370–373.

Harrington, H., and Theis, C. Institutional factors perceived by baccalaureate graduates as influencing their performance as staff nurses. *Nursing Research*, June 1968, *17*, 228–235.

Hegedus, K. S. The Volicer Hospital Stress Rating Scale: A patient outcome criterion measure. *Supervisor Nurse*, January 1979, *10*, 40–45.

Hodgman, E. C. Closing the gap between research and practice: Changing the answers to the Who, the Where, and the How of nursing research. *International Journal of Nursing Studies*, 1979, *16*, 105–110.

Hodgman, E. C. Student research in service agencies. *Nursing Outlook*, September 1978, *26*, 558–565.

Hegyvary, S. Foundations of primary nursing. *Nursing Clinics of North America*, June 1977, *12*, 185–196.

Hegyvary, S., and Haussman, R. Monitoring nursing care quality. *Journal of Nursing Administration*, November 1976, *6*, 3–37.

Henderson, C. Can nursing care hasten recovery? *American Journal of Nursing*, June 1964, *64*, 80–83.

HEW. Health Education Primary Nursing: Can It Improve Patient Education? Bureau of Health Education under HEW Contract No. 200-75-0542, Center for Disease Control, Bureau of Health Education, Community Program Development Division, Atlanta, Ga., 1977.

Hymovich, D. How children, mothers, and nurses view primary and team nursing. *American Journal of Nursing*, November 1980. *80*, 2041–2045.

Hymovich, D. P. The effects of primary nursing care on children's parents and nurses' perceptions of the pediatric nursing role. *Nursing Research Report*, May 1977, *12*, 7.

Isler, C. Rx for a sick hospital: Primary nursing care. *RN*, February 1976, pp. 60–65. (Also see p. 67 for "Comments for 'Rx for a Sick Hospital: Primary Nursing Care.' ")

Jennings, C. P. Primary care and the question of obsolescence. *Journal of Psychiatric Nursing*, January 1977, *15*, 9–17.

Johnson, M., and Martin, H. A sociological analysis of the nurse role. *American Journal of Nursing*, February 1958, *58*, 373–377.

Jones, K. Study documents effect of primary nursing on renal transplant patients. *Hospitals JAHA*, December 1975, *49*, 85–89.

Katz, D., and Kahn, R. Open systems theory. In Grusky, O., and Miller, G., *The Sociology of Organizations*. New York: The Free Press, 1970.

Katz, F. Nurses. In A. Etzioni, (Ed.). *The Semi-Professions and Their Organization*. New York: The Free Press, 1969.

Keane, Vera R. What are the challenges—the major elements of primary nursing care? *Hospital Topics*, November–December 1974, p. 43–46.

Keiser, G. J., and Bickle, I. M. Attitude change as a motivational factor. *Nursing Research*, September–October 1980, *29*, 290–294.

Knecht, A. Innovation of four tower west: Why? *American Journal of Nursing*, May 1973, *73*, 808–810.

Kramer, M. Team nursing—a means or an end? *Nursing Outlook*, October 1971, *19*, 648–652.

Lambertsen, E. *Education for Nursing Leadership*. Philadelphia: J. B. Lippincott Co., 1958.

Leonard, M. Health issues and primary nursing in nephrology care. *Nursing Clinics of North America*, September 1975, *10*, 413–420.

Lindeman, C. Measuring quality of nursing care: Part One. *Journal of Nursing Administration*, June 1976, *6*, 7–9.

Lindeman, C. Measuring quality of nursing care: Part Two. *Journal of Nursing Administration*, September 1976, *6*, 19–23.

Logsdon, A. Why primary nursing? *Nursing Clinics of North America*, June 1973, *8*, 283–291.

Maas, M., Specht, J., and Jacox, A. Nurse autonomy, reality not rhetoric. *American Journal of Nursing*, December 1975, *75*, 2201–2205.

Manfredi, C. Primary nursing and change: A case study. *Nursing Leadership*, September 1980, *3*, 8–15.

Manthey, M. A theoretical framework for primary nursing. *Journal of Nursing Administration*, June 1980, *10*, 11–15.

Manthey, M. If you are instituting primary nursing. *American Journal of Nursing*, March 1978, *78*, 426.

Manthey, M. Primary nursing is alive and well in the hospital. *American Journal of Nursing*, January 1973, *73*, 83–87.

Manthey, M. *The Practice of Primary Nursing*, Boston: Blackwell Scientific Publications, Inc., 1980, pp. 1–96.

Manthey, M., et al. Primary nursing workshop. Audio Cassettes 1-2, United Hospital, Inc., St. Paul, Minnesota, 1974.

Manthey, M., Ciske, K., Robertson, P., and Harris, I. Primary nursing: A return to the concept of "My Nurse" and "My Patient." *Nursing Forum*, Winter 1970, *9*, 60–84.

Manthey, M., and Kramer, M. A dialogue on primary nursing. *Nursing Forum*, September 1970, *9*, 356–379.

Marram, G. Innovation on Four Tower West: What happened? *American Journal of Nursing*, May 1973, *73*, 814–815.

Marram, G. D. Patients' evaluation of their care: Importance to the nurse. *Nursing Outlook*, May 1973, *21*, 322–324.

Marram, G. The comparative costs of operating a team and primary nursing unit. *Journal of Nursing Administration*, May 1976, *6*, 21–24.

Marram, G., et al. *Cost Effectiveness of Primary and Team Nursing*, Wakefield, Mass.: Contemporary Publishing, Inc., 1976.

Marram, G., et al. *Primary Nursing: A Model for Individualized Care*, St. Louis, Mo.: The C. V. Mosby Co., 1974.

Marram, G., Schlegel, M., and Bevis, E. *Primary Nursing: A Model for Individualized Care*. St. Louis: The C. V. Mosby Co., 1974.

Medaglia, M. A coronary care unit implements primary nursing. *Canadian Nurse*, May 1978, *74*, 32–32.

Mauksch, I. Prescription for survival. *American Journal of Nursing*, December 1972, *72*, 2189–2193.

Mayer, G., and Bailey, K. Adapting the patient care conference to primary nursing. *Journal of Nursing Administration*, June 1979, *IX:6*, 7–10.

McCarthy, D., and Schifalacqua. Primary nursing: Its implementation and six month outcome. *Journal of Nursing Administration*, May 1978, *8*, 29–32. (Also see *Journal of Nursing Administration*, August 1978, for readers' reactions.)

McGreevy, M. E., and Coates, M. L. Primary nursing implementation using the project nurse and the nursing process framework. *Journal of Nursing Administration*, February 1980, pp. 9–15.

Metzer, N. *The Health Care Supervisor's Handbook*. Germantown: Md.: Aspen Publications, 1978.

Miller, D. Education for nursing service administration. *Nursing Forum*, 1968, *7*, 375–385.

Montag, M. The Education of Nursing Technicians. New York: G. P. Putnam's Sons, 1951.

Moritz, D. A. Primary nursing: Implications for curriculum development. *Journal of Nursing Education*, March 1979, *18*, 33–37.

Mundinger, M. Primary nursing: Impact on the education department. *Nursing Outlook*, October 1973, *21*, 69–77.

Mundinger, M. Primary nurse—role evolution. *Nursing Outlook*, October 1973, *21*, 642–645.

Nenner, V. C., Curtis, E. M., and Eckhoff, C. M. Primary nursing. *Supervisor Nurse*, May 1977, *8*, 14–16.

National League for Nursing. *Primary Nursing—One Nurse, One Client Planning Care Together*. New York: NLN Pub. No. 52–1695, 1977: (a) Ferguson, V. Primary nursing—a modality of care for today. (b) Russell, R. Rationale for primary nursing care. (c) Marram, G. Principles and processes in instituting the change to primary nursing. (d) O'Leary, J. Primary nursing care: Implementing change. (e) Mobley, N. Confrontation of the incongruities between theory and practice. (f) O'Leary, J. Organizational structure and role responsibilities. (g) Russell, R. Process and implementation—attitudes and approaches.

National League for Nursing. *The Realities of Primary Nursing Care—Risk,*

*Roles, Research*. New York: NLN Pub. No. 52-1716, 1978: (a) Donaho, B. What are the risks of change? (b) Copp, L. Building decisions on data. (c) Perry, E. Needed changes in education. (d) Salyer, J., and Sloan, R. Bridging the gap between education and service. (e) Rye, D. From dreams to reality. (f) Durham, R. A plan for researching the effects of primary nursing care. (g) Wisener, S. Role changes in primary nursing. (h) Nichols, P. Primary nursing in the Mt. Olive Family Medicine Center. (i) Jefferson, C. Primary nursing in a short-term pediatric setting. (j) Selleck, C. Primary nursing in a hematology unit.

National League of Nursing Education. *A Curriculum for Schools of Nursing: A Report Prepared by the Committee on Education*. New York: National League of Nursing Education, 1927.

National League of Nursing Education. *A Study on the Use of the Graduate Nurse for Bedside Nursing in the Hospital: A Report Prepared by the Department of Studies*. New York: National League of Nursing Education, 1933.

National League of Nursing Education. *Standard Curriculum for Schools of Nursing: A Report Prepared by the Committee on Education*. Baltimore: Waverly Press, 1917.

Norris, C. Delusions that trap nurses. *Nursing Outlook*, January 1973, *21*, 18–21.

Notter, L., and Spalding, E. *Professional Nursing: Foundations, Perspectives, and Relationships* (9th ed.). New York: J. B. Lippincott Co., 1976.

Ojeda, M. Primary nursing for shortened stay surgical patients. *Supervisor Nurse*, September 1976, pp. 42, 45, 48.

O'Leary, J., and Hill, E. Staffing a primary nursing unit. *Nursing Administration Quarterly*, Summer 1977, *1*, 69–78.

Olsen, A. Change takes time. *Supervisor Nurse*, September 1976, pp. 51–59.

Osinski, E., and Powals, J. The cost of all RN staffed primary nursing. *Supervisor Nurse*, January 1980, pp. 16–21.

Page, M. Primary nursing: Perceptions of a head nurse. *American Journal of Nursing*, August 1974, *74*, 1435–1436.

Passos, J. Accountability: Myth or mandate? *Journal of Nursing Administration*, Vol. 3, May–June 1973.

Peplau, H. Professional closeness. *Nursing Forum*, Vol. 8, 1969.

Pisani, S. H. Primary nursing: Aftermath of change. *Nursing Administration Quarterly*, Winter 1977, pp. 107–113.

Pohl, M. *Teaching Function of the Nursing Practitioner*. Dubuque, Iowa: William Brown, Co., 1968.

Prendergast, J. Implementing problem oriented records in a primary nursing system. *Nursing Clinics of North America*, June 1977, *12*, 235–246.

Previte, V. J. Continuing care in a primary nursing setting: Role of a clinical specialist. *International Nursing Review*, March–April 1979, *26*, 53–56.

Primary nursing. *Nursing Clinics of North America*, Vol. 12, Special Edition, September 1977.

Probst, J., and Noga, J. A decentralized nursing care delivery system. *Supervisor Nurse*, January 1980, pp. 57–60.

Pryma, R. Primary nursing—a working philosophy—an organizational style. *The Magazine*. Chicago: Rush-Presbyterian–St. Luke's Medical Center, Spring 1978.

Putt, A. The nurse educator looks at the nurse clinician. *Military Medicine*, January 1977, *142*, 45–57.

Rieve, J. Primary nursing in a psychiatric inpatient setting. *Alumni Magazine*, 1974, *73*, 20–21.

Risser, N. L. Development of an instrument to measure patient satisfaction with nurses and nursing care in primary care settings. *Nursing Research*, 1975, *24*, 45.

Robinson, A. Primary nurse: Specialist in total care. *RN*, April 1974, pp. 31–35.

Romero, M., and Lewis, G. Patient and staff perceptions as a basis for change. *Nursing Clinics of North America*, June 1977, *12*, 197–203.

Schlegel, M. W. Innovation on Four Tower West: How? *American Journal of Nursing*, 1973, *73*, 811–813.

Schorr, T. Let's hear it for primary nursing (editorial). *American Journal of Nursing*, November 1977.

Schultz, R., and Johnson, A. *Management of Hospitals*, New York: McGraw-Hill, 1976.

Schwab, Sister M. . . . Where nurses' aides don't do all the nursing care . . . *Journal of Gerontological Nursing*, May–June 1976, *2*, 20–23.

Smith, C. C. Primary nursing care—a substantive nursing care delivery system. *Nursing Administration Quarterly*, Winter 1977.

Sobczak, C. L. Pharmacy and primary nursing: Potential for conflict and cooperation. *Nursing Administration Quarterly*, Winter 1977.

Spitzer, R. Making primary nursing work. *Supervisor Nurse*, January 1979, pp. 12–14.

Spilotro, S. A unified role in nursing. *Nursing Administration*, Part I:21, Spring 1979.

Spoth, J. Primary nursing: The agony and the ecstasy. *Nursing Clinics of North America*, June 1977, *12*, 211–234.

Stevens, B. The problems in nursing's middle management. *Journal of Nursing Administration*, September–October 1974, *4*, p. 37.

Stuvert, N. Nothing is as permanent as change. *Nation's Business*, August 1959, *47*, 33, 57–59.

Vanservellen, G. M. Primary nursing—the adoption of a nursing care modality. *Nursing and Health Care*, October 1980, pp. 144–149.

Watts, V., and O'Leary, J. Ten components of primary nursing. *Nursing Dimensions*, Winter 1980, VIII, 90–95.

Werner, J., and Evanston Hospital Staff, The Evanston Story: Primary nursing comes alive. *Nursing Research*, September–October 1974, *24*, 9–50.

Williams, L. Evaluation of nursing care: A primary nursing project, Part I. *Supervisor Nurse*, January 1975, pp. 32–39.

Wolff, K. Change: Implementation of primary nursing through ad hocracy. *Journal of Nursing Administration*, December 1977.

Young, J. P., Giovannetti, P. B., and Lewison, D. *A Comparative Study of Team and Primary Nursing Care on Two Surgical Inpatient Units*. Division of Nursing, Bureau of Health Manpower Health Resources Administration, Department of Health, Education and Welfare, Contract No. HRA 232-78-0150, June 1980.

Young, J. P., Giovannetti, P. B., Lewison, D., and Thomas, M. L. *Factors Affecting Nurse Staffing in Acute Hospitals: A Review and Critique of the Literature*. Division of Nursing, Bureau of Health Manpower, Health Resources Administration, Department of Health and Human Services, Contract. No. HRA 232-78-0150, September 1980.

Yura, H., Ozimek, D., and Walsh, M. *Nursing Leadership: Theory and Process*, New York: Appleton-Century-Crofts, 1976.

Zander, K. *Primary Nursing: Development and Management*, Germantown, Md.: Aspen Systems Corporation, 1980.

Zander, K. S. Primary nursing won't work . . . unless the head nurse lets it. *The Journal of Nursing Administration*, October 1977, 7, 19–23.

# Index

Absence from duty, 73, 74
Absolute standard in evaluation, 70–71
Administrative assistant, job description, 86
American Nurses' Association, 38
American Society of Superintendents of Training Schools for Nurses, 14
Apprenticeship training, 13, 18
Assignments, 73, 74
Assistant director, 10. *See also* Middle manager
Authority, 32
decentralization of, 59

Baccalaureate programs in nursing, 19–20, 120
deficits in, 93–95
primary nursing and middle management, 99–102
Basic Leadership/Management Course in Clinical Setting, 108–111
Bellevue Training School, N.Y.C., 13
Boston Training School, 13
Bulletin boards, uses of, 52–53

Case patient care delivery system, 3–5
Change process
impatience with, 87–88
utilization of, 60–65
Client-centered health care philosophy, 23–28

Clinical skills, application of, 16, 40–42
Cognitive knowledge, application of, 40–42
Collegiate Schools of Nursing, 16
Committee of the Functions of Nursing, 18
Communication skills, in management, 51–56
Connecticut Training School, New Haven, 13
Consultant role, 33, 35, 59
Consumer-oriented health care philosophy, 23–28
Contracts
implementing, 73–75
negotiating, 72–73
Controlling, in managerial process, 50–51
Coordination of care, 6
Coordinator, nursing clinical, 78–85. *See also* Middle manager
Courses. *See also* Education and primary nursing
leadership/management, 108–113
patient care delivery via primary nursing, 113–114

Decentralization, 59, 89
Delegation, in management, 43
Director of Nursing Services, 27, 95. *See also* Top management

**DATE DUE**

| | | | |
|---|---|---|---|
| 4/18 TS | | | |
| 3/25 em | | | |
| 5/6 R | | | |
| | | | |
| | | | |
| | | | |
| | | | |
| | | | |